1. The Unlikely Friendship

   - A heartwarming tale of an unexpected bond between a lonely elderly man and a stray cat.

2. The Magical Library

   - A story about a library that holds books with magical properties, bringing joy and wonder to its readers.

3. A Journey Through Time

   - A time-traveling adventure where a young scientist discovers the secrets of the past and future.

4. The Enchanted Forest

   - An exploration of a mysterious forest where magical creatures and unexpected friendships await.

5. The Lost Star

   - A cosmic journey as a young girl embarks on a mission to save a fallen star and restore its light to the sky.

6. The Curious Case of Mr. Puddlewick

   - A whimsical mystery involving a peculiar detective and a town baffled by strange occurrences.

7. Pixel Crush: My VR Date with Destiny

   - A virtual reality love story that unfolds in the world of gaming, proving that connections can transcend digital boundaries.

8. Houston, We Have a Problem: How Sally Saved the Day

   - An astronaut's tale of quick thinking and resourcefulness to overcome a critical situation in space.

9. A Deadline to Meet

   - The story of a freelance writer facing an impossible deadline, and finding inspiration in unexpected places.

10. A Royal Feast to Remember

   - A chef's unexpected opportunity to cook for the royal palace, filled with challenges and triumphs.

11. Riding the Monster Wave

   - A surfer's daring encounter with a colossal wave and the friendship that becomes the key to his survival.

12. A Lesson in Likes

   - A heartwarming story of a young boy teaching his elderly neighbor about social media, connecting generations.

13. A Family's Love

- A tale of siblings setting aside differences to care for their ailing mother, finding strength in family bonds.

14. A Helping Paw and a New Lease on Life

- The story of a shy man's transformative journey sparked by rescuing an injured dog, leading to newfound confidence.

15. When Grandma Gets a Handmade Gift

- A charming narrative of grandchildren crafting heartfelt gifts for their grandma, showcasing the beauty of handmade gestures.

Title: "Mittens' Mischievous Cookie Caper"

It was a sunlit Saturday afternoon, and little Sally found herself immersed in the delightful world of baking chocolate chip cookies with her mom. "These smell delicious!" exclaimed Sally as she delicately took the first batch out of the oven.

Just as the aroma wafted through the air, their mischievous cat, Mittens, strolled into the kitchen, captivated by the irresistible scent. "Meow," said Mittens, casting Sally an irresistible gaze. "I think she wants a cookie," chuckled Sally. However, Mom intervened, "No, Mittens! Cookies are not suitable for kitties. You'll get your cat food in a little bit."

Undeterred, Mittens retreated, her dejection overshadowed by a sneaky plan forming in her feline mind. When Mom and Sally left the kitchen to enjoy a movie, Mittens seized the opportunity. She leaped onto the counter with stealthy grace and devoured a whole cookie in one swift bite. "So good!" thought Mittens.

But after finishing the first cookie, Mittens started to feel a little peculiar. Her tummy grumbled and rumbled. "Meow!" she yowled, leaping down. In her haste, she accidentally knocked over the entire platter of cookies!

Crumb by crumb, they scattered across the kitchen floor. Mittens attempted to gather them up but only conformed her fur with crumbs. At that moment, Sally walked back in. "Oh no!" cried Sally. "What happened to my cookies?!"

She glared at Mittens, who put on her best innocent face. However, Sally wasn't fooled. "You naughty kitty!" Sally scolded. "I told you cookies aren't for cats. Now look at the mess!" Mittens hung her head, feeling a pang of shame.

Sally's anger quickly transformed into concern. "Mom!" she called. "I think Mittens' tummy hurts from eating the cookies. What do we do?" Mom hurried in and scooped up the guilty-looking Mittens. Sure enough, her belly was swollen, emitting loud gurgles.

After a visit to the veterinarian and some special medicine, Mittens began to feel better. She had certainly learned her lesson about swiping human food without permission! As for the cookies, with some teamwork, Sally and Mom managed to scrape up most of the crumbs and assemble a new batch, just in time for the neighborhood kids coming over for a playdate. Mittens received extra cuddles for being such a good patient during her recovery. The end!

Title: "Pawsome Bonds: Lyla's Unlikely Birthday Bash"

It was Lyla the dog's 12th birthday, and her owners Mike and Sarah were hosting an extravagant party in her honor. Adorned with a green party hat featuring balloons and surrounded by her favorite toys, Lyla eagerly awaited the festivities, not to mention the grand dog cake with peanut butter icing.

Lyla's canine companions from the neighborhood—Rocky with his distinctive spots, the fluffy Snowball, and the energetic Buddy—filled the backyard with joy as they engaged in a lively game of fetch. However, the celebration took an unexpected turn when a scruffy tomcat named Smokey leaped over the fence.

"Hey, what's going on here?" inquired Smokey. The dogs erupted into a chorus of barks. "It's a party, but cats aren't invited!" declared Rocky.

Approaching Smokey, Lyla explained, "It's my birthday. But my mom and dad only invited dogs. I'm sorry, Smokey, but you'll have to leave." Smokey hung his head dejectedly.

At that moment, Mike emerged. "What's all the ruckus about?" he questioned. Spotting Smokey, he empathized with the lonely cat. "You know, it wouldn't hurt to have one cat at this dog party," Mike suggested to Lyla.

Gasps filled the air, but Lyla wagged her tail happily. Smokey's eyes lit up as Mike handed him a slice of cake. Soon, dogs and cats alike were engaged in games like Pin the Tail on the Dog and Musical Bumps.

As the day drew to a close, Smokey had not only made new dog friends but also discovered that dogs weren't as bad as he had thought. "Thanks for letting me crash your party, Lyla!" expressed Smokey as he prepared to depart. However, Mike and Sarah sensed Smokey's homelessness.

"What do you say we adopt this stray cat?" Mike proposed to Lyla, who barked in agreement. Thus, Smokey became part of their family, emerging as Lyla's new best friend. Their story illustrated that with kindness, dogs, and cats could forge meaningful friendships. It was the best birthday ever for Lyla and the beginning of a beautiful interspecies camaraderie.

Title: "Rocky's Nuggets Adventure: Lessons in Canine Caution"

On a sunny Saturday afternoon, young Jimmy found himself at his grandma's house, eagerly anticipating a lunch of his favorite—chicken nuggets. "I'm making your favorite - chicken nuggets for lunch!" announced Grandma, igniting Jimmy's hunger.

As the nuggets baked in the oven, Grandma's excitable terrier Rocky sensed the irresistible aroma wafting through the house. The terrier, overcome with excitement, began pacing back and forth in the kitchen, drooling in anticipation. Seizing a moment when Grandma stepped away, Rocky saw his chance.

With a leap, he nudged the oven door open, only to recoil as the heat hit him. "Yip!" cried Rocky, jumping back and accidentally sending the entire sheet of nuggets tumbling onto the floor. Nugget chaos ensued as they scattered across the tiles, and Rocky attempted to devour as many as he could.

Grandma returned, witnessing the aftermath. "No, Rocky!" she scolded, but the nuggets were already everywhere. Rocky, with nugget crumbs falling from his mouth, hung his head. Grandma sighed, realizing the predicament. "Now how am I supposed to feed Jimmy?"

Enter Jimmy, who entered the kitchen asking, "Where are my nuggets?" His joy turned to tears as he saw the mess. Grandma comforted him while Rocky, with a guilty expression, retreated to the porch, tail between his legs.

Grandma knew she had to remedy the situation quickly before Jimmy's hunger turned into hungriness. Swiftly, she whipped up a new batch of nuggets in the microwave, saturating the kitchen with their savory aroma once again.

Jimmy's tears ceased as the enticing scent reached him. As they savored the nuggets, Grandma had an idea. "Rocky looks sad out there. I think he deserves one nugget as a lesson learned." Surprisingly, she tossed him a treat through the window.

Rocky gobbled it up and expressed his remorse with a lick of Grandma's hand. All was forgiven, and Rocky became more cautious around food from that day on. As for Jimmy, with a satisfied stomach, he resumed playing, having learned that not all problems have to end in tears.

Title: "Mittens' Pizza Adventure: A Tale of Crispy Crust and Second Chances"

On a Friday night, the air buzzing with excitement, little Susie was having a sleepover with her best friend Emma. "I can't wait for pizza and movies!" exclaimed Susie. Their anticipations soared as the doorbell rang, announcing the arrival of their long-awaited pizza.

While Susie's mom paid the delivery guy, the mischievous tabby cat, Mittens, detected the heavenly pizza aroma. Her tummy rumbled in response. Seizing the opportunity when no one was looking, Mittens stealthily approached and nudged the steaming pizza box open with her paw.

"Mmm, cheese!" thought Mittens, taking a bold bite of a slice. Alas, the pizza was hot! "Yeowch!" cried Mittens, leaping back and unintentionally sending the entire pizza onto the floor. As slices scattered, Mittens attempted to devour as much evidence as possible.

Susie and Emma entered the room, exclaiming, "Where's the pizza?!?" Spotting Mittens with sauce-coated whiskers, Susie quickly deduced what had occurred. "You pizza pirate!" scolded Susie, while Mittens meowed innocently.

With the original pizza now a casualty, the girls faced the dilemma of what to eat. As Susie started to cry, her mom came to the rescue with a creative solution. "We still have pizza leftovers from last night in the fridge," she suggested, promptly microwaving them.

Even as the crisped edges wafted their enticing aroma, Mittens' tummy rumbled once again. Susie's mom tossed Mittens a small piece with a laugh. "Next time, ask before sampling the goods!" From that day on, Mittens learned to keep her paws off human food unless invited.

The moral of the story? Crying over spilled pizza won't solve anything. Through creativity and kindness between critters and kids, even the messiest of mix-ups can end with full tummies and new laughs to share.

Title: "Laughter Among the Leaves: The Tale of the Treehouse Treasure"

In Johnny's backyard, nestled within the branches of a majestic oak tree, stood the treehouse that he and his best friend Sally cherished. Constructed with the helping hands of Johnny's dad, it served as a haven for their summertime adventures.

One day, the spirit of adventure struck Johnny, and he proposed, "Let's have a treasure hunt!" Excitement filled the air as he revealed his plan to hide some of his favorite toys and candy around the treehouse for Sally to discover.

Johnny gathered his prized possessions - a bag of gummy bears, action figures, and his beloved baseball card collection. Together, they were carefully placed in a box to serve as the treasure chest. The treasure hunt commenced, with Johnny strategically hiding clues and snacks in cunning spots, such as inside an old boot and beneath the floorboards.

As Johnny completed the last hiding place, disaster struck. The treasure chest proved too heavy, and as he set it down, the aging treehouse floorboards gave way with a resounding CRACK. Down tumbled Johnny and the chest, crashing through branches until they reached the ground below.

From above, Sally cried out in panic, "Johnny, are you okay?!" Miraculously, Johnny, though scraped and dusty, was unharmed. However, the treasure chest had burst open, scattering its contents everywhere.

Johnny's mom, drawn outside by the commotion, first adopted a stern expression but soon burst into laughter. "I guess the floor just couldn't handle all that treasure!" she chuckled. Johnny, joining in the laughter, realized the humor in the situation. Together, they cleaned up the delightful mess.

The moral of the story? A treehouse filled with toys and treats is delightful, but the true treasures lie in laughter and the company of friends.

Title: "Jane's Corner Cafe: Brewing Community Bonds"

In the heart of the neighborhood, Jane's Corner Cafe stood as a daily gathering place, emanating the irresistible aroma of freshly brewed coffee that drew in the regular crowd seeking their daily fix.

Harold, the local mailman, was the first to arrive, greeted by Jane with his usual ham and egg sandwich paired with an extra-strong cup of joe. The flower shop's Linda followed, bringing colorful blossoms to brighten up the cafe as she chatted with Harold over banana nut muffins.

Before the morning rush, Sam, the professor from the nearby university, made his pitstop, engaging his analytical mind with dense texts while enjoying oatmeal and orange juice.

As the morning crowd poured in, a diverse array of patrons found comfort in Jane's comforting cuisine and upbeat company. Bustling businessmen, harried moms, and retirees all reveled in the camaraderie of Jane's Cafe.

Some regulars preferred quiet moments, while others engaged in lively conversations. Wendy, the rec center enthusiast, shared updates with Barbara the librarian. Steve, the postal worker, animatedly recounted tales from his route to anyone who would listen over crepes.

The retiree table became a central hub, where the witty Robert held court with wild stories from his adventurous past. Betty, Henry, and others formed a close-knit family within these walls.

Through it all, Jane played the role of glue, keeping spirits high with her energetic bustling, and warm smiles. Whether someone needed a kind ear or a hot refill, Jane ensured that everyone left satisfied.

As midday arrived, the crowd thinned, but a core group remained, continuing their conversations, solving puzzles, and reading. Amidst changing lives, Jane's Corner Cafe remained a constant, reminder of the things that truly matter—community, camaraderie, and breaking bread together with neighbors both old and new.

Title: "Jane's Corner Cafe Chronicles: The Case of the Missing Banana Cake"

At 7 am on a leisurely Saturday, Jane's Corner Cafe was just stirring, providing a brief lull for cleanup. Jane diligently wiped down counters, Harold wielded a broom, and Linda fluffed pillows with care.

Unexpectedly, the door swung open, ushering in a gust of wind. In stumbled Sally, the postal worker, clutching a sodden package—victim to an unexpected downpour during the morning mail delivery.

"Help yourself to dry clothes," Jane offered, guiding the shivering Sally to a chair by the fireplace. Sally's drenched cargo, including the morning mail, socks, and boots, sprawled out to dry.

Soon, Jane's keen sense of smell led her to the lost parcel's contents—an entire banana cake intended for the upcoming bake sale. Unfortunately, one small, waterlogged box held nothing but a soggy mess of crumbs.

Determined to unveil the cake bandit, Jane rallied the regulars. "We've got a mystery on our hands, and our treats are missing. Let's put our wits to work!" Harold suspected squirrels, Linda thought birds, while Sam remained undisturbed, snoozing in the face of intrigue.

Their first clue emerged in the form of purring—Kit, the cafe cat, was found licking creamy paws beside the remnants of the telltale box. But could a feline be the culprit for cake thievery? Perplexed, Wendy recalled a recent observation.

Just the day before, Wendy spotted mischievous raccoons near the bins, one of them washing something yellow and gooey. The gang followed Wendy's lead into the alley, discovering two satisfied masked bandits behind the last bin, bellies bulging!

With the case resolved, the raccoons were left to rest peacefully. Back inside, Linda whipped up a new cake "for a good cause," and Sam rejuvenated with a cup of coffee. The kooky crew soon indulged in the morning's shenanigans, reveling in sweets well-earned. Another mystery was solved, all thanks to the eccentric charms of Jane's Corner Cafe.

Title: "The Fantastical Fairy Festival Fiasco: A Whimsical Woodland Tale"

Deep within the enchanted Fairy Forest, a vibrant buzz filled the colorful glade as fairy folk gathered for their annual festival—a whimsical weekend of wonder, magic, and mirth.

Tinker Bell flitted about, preparing prismatic pixie dust potions and sprinkling shimmering stardust on mushroom seats and daisy decor. Butterflies fluttered flags of fluttering fins and fibers between fir and fungus folks.

Queen Clarion called the commencing ceremonies to order with a cheerful chime of crystal. The woodland wild poured past pelting paddocks to their patterned placements, eagerly anticipating the festivities. However, unbeknownst to the united undergrowth's upstanding upholders, unexpected events were about to unfold.

The first signs struck during the songful singing salutations. A rogue rabbit rushed through, recklessly rampaging amongst revelers, releasing repellent roots and remains in its panicked passing.

An uproar ensued as fouled fairies fled the fetid fumes. Fairy Mary attempted appeasement, but futility found further frustrations mounting. Wounded woodlanders writhed and wailed, and worry grew about how to expunge the calamity.

Jubilant jester Jax skipped onto the scene with a solution sent straight from sparkling serendipity. He seized the sadly suffering bunny with a bound and performed a purifying procedure, producing pleasing progress. Peace prevailed once more upon the populace.

However, further farces followed fast without fail. Festival fires flickered and then inexplicably ignited into an unstoppable inferno. Flames fled across ferns and flourished forest features near and far. All seemed lost in smoke and sorrow when mystifying mists miraculously materialized, dousing devastation with divine deliverance.

In the twilight hours, the fatigued fairies' festival fervor found a fresh resurgence, with dancing and dining resuming delightfully. Tales of the day's turmoil would traverse the treetops for times to come, bringing bursts of bright banter and mirthful memories to last through fall and winter waiting. Thus, the fantastical festival freak frenzy faded fondly into fairy folklore folk fame.

Title: "The Picnic Pantry Predicament: A Culinary Catastrophe and Friendly Flourishes"

On a sunny Saturday, Betty buzzed with activity, meticulously packing baskets of bread, berries, and biscuits for the community center's cookout. As the head of the food committee, she prided herself on providing prompt and palatable provisions.

While folding flavorful flatbreads, Friendly Frank, the florist, arrived, bringing with him fragrant floral fresheners to enhance the fantastic feast. He announced his arrival, carrying cheerful cascades of carnations.

Betty, beaming before the bright bouquets bursting with color, agreed, "These viburnums and verbenas will spruce up any spread for sure." However, arranging the aromatic additions proved arduous, accidentally activating an obscure object.

Amidst the commotion, a curious cube had been casually cast aside—a vintage valuables vacillator designed to vanish unwanted items with a push of its magic malachite button. As Betty battled bursting baskets, her elbow accidentally hit its devilish switch.

Before their bewildered eyes, all provisions promptly presented precipitated into pure pandemonium! Picnic preparations seemingly dissipated into a darkening mist. Betty broke down blubbering in despair, certain she had destroyed their delicious dinner duties.

However, Friendly Frank, ever the cool-headed companion, caught a familiar flicker from the empty cube's cryptic carvings. With well-wishing words and a wave, he whisked away the object, willing the vanished victuals to reappear at once.

True to his talent for transference, the erstwhile eats revived right where they rightfully belonged. Betty bleated with brightened blessings, thanking her trusted compatriot. Thanks to fast friendship, another food fiasco faced deft defusing, and the picnic prophesied a palate-pleasing party after all.

Title: "The Grand Garden Gala Mystery: A Bountiful Bake-Off and a Whimsical Whodunit"

The annual Garden Gala was fast approaching, and Betty, the brilliant baker behind the bustling botanical bashes, was busy baking batches of blissful brownies, bundt cakes, and biscotti for the big botany bonanza. Her goal this year was to dazzle with decadent desserts more than ever before, infusing her almonds with ambrosial orange zest and indulging in fudgy frostings flecked with flakes of 24-karat gold.

As the gala's glorious day dawned, volunteers added final flourishes, filling every flat surface with fresh flowers and adorning the lush landscape with a resplendent rainbow of ricocheting reflections. Bunches of balloons bounced gaily as banners announced the best in blooms.

Betty's bountiful baked beauties, beautifully boxed, were lined up to be unveiled later. However, as the festivities began, something seemed strangely serene. Strolling guests grew gradually grave, grumbling about missing merrymakers and a lack of lively laughter typically tickling their taste buds.

A quick headcount revealed the conundrum—none of the committee's key members could be found! Linda, the festival leader, was noticeably absent, as were party planners Polly and Priscilla. Baffled Betty took charge, attempting to track the truant troop with walkie-talkies to no avail.

Frantic phone calls provided few facts, forcing volunteers to venture bravely on barricading their worry for now. As the afternoon ambled ahead aimlessly without answers, agitation arose amongst the ambling attendees.

Just then, a jittery Junior Jenny hurried over, out of breath but bearing a bizarre befuddling bulletin. She excitedly explained discovering a crumpled clue crammed into a carefully concealed cache amidst the carnations! All huddled close, heart rates heightening, as the missive was recited:

"If floral fans hope to find our frolicking flock with fleet feet, follow clues left in landscaping to our lurking locale posthaste! First riddle: We shine so sunny where lilies lie low and lilacs lift leaves long. Look lively, the next are nearby! - The Missing Members"

After hours of hassle, at least they had a hopeful hunt ahead! Teams took turns traversing the terraced terrain, adeptly answering each enigma until victoriously glimpsing the vanished VIPs safe and sound ahead. The mischief had been a prank to promote pride in their prized plant paradise. Betty breathed a big sigh of relief that her bountiful baked beauties could at last be boldly brought forth! Their grand day, once in doubt, now danced delightfully onward with no dreary drips to dampen their dazzling display remaining. All present parted with memories to last, content the confusion had culminated completely convivially in the end!

Title: "The Whimsical World of Widgets: A Tale of Enchanted Inventions and Unexpected Adventure"

Deep in the enchanted forest, hidden amongst twisting treetops, lay a curious kingdom oft overlooked by outsiders. Inside a sprawling willow's winding way grew a glimmering gateway welcoming all to the whimsical world within - Widget Woods!

This fanciful realm was ruled capably by the benevolent Baroness Willow, a wise witch of 800 winters whose magic kept things whirring. She took pride in her people, a chipper clan of quirky craftsfolk called Widgets. Using wondrous witchery, these woodland workers wove countless contraptions more curious each day.

From cog-powered carriages to self-stringing harps, no invention was too implausible for these innovative individuals. With works centered around their bustling burg's beating heart - the Bazaar of Bright Builds. Here the Widgets would debut their dazzling devices, proudly presenting peculiar products to please both practical and playful patrons.

Each eve, Baroness Willow would wander through the rows, reviewing and rewarding the day's exceptional efforts. One fateful fortnight, she stumbled upon two stand-out submissions sure to spark smiles. Young Wren had designed delicate dreamcatchers that danced to dreamy melodies when moonbeams shone through.

And eccentric Erik unveiled his "Electronic Experience Enhancer" - a curiously conical contraption meant to magnify mundane moments into memories marvelous. Both creations were commended, and Erik pledged to debut his device at the upcoming celebration - the Whimsical Widget Weekend Wonder!

Come festivities, the forest filled up quickly. Food and frolic filled the fields while special showcases dazzled in the square. Erik unveiled his device, a mesmerizing sight that scattered sparkles and spun sound into shimmering scenes when activated.

Yet as wonder washed over onlookers, odd occurrences began. Every eerie enactment ended eventually, leaving watchers troubled and tired when typically tittering. With each show, the effects seemed to escalate, draining more dear souls of spirit and laughter.

The Baroness was alarmed, confronting Erik at once. Inside she found his invention inexplicably infected, intentions inverted! Magic went mad meant to mar merriment now, not augment it. Together they contrived a countercharm, containing the corruption with care. Calamity ceased; cheer restored - thanks to their teamwork tandems!

In time, the people returned to themselves, memories mended and mysteries explained once more. Erik learned a valuable lesson on limits that lingered long. And thus another quirky quest in Widget Woods concluded blithely that day! The kingdom kept whirring warmly as before.

Title: "Whimsical Wood's Carnival of Curiosities: A Tale of Quirky Creatures and Marvelous Mayhem"

Deep in the magical Whimsical Wood, the eccentric elves and industrious imps were making marvelous preparations for their annual Carnival of Curiosities! Under the watchful eye of Fairy Queen Willow, orders were fluttering - set up the stages, string up the streamers, stoke the fairy fires to welcome wandering wanderlusts from far and wide!

One industrious elf was especially invested - Edmund the inventor. Since last year's event, he'd spent hours developing his most outlandish idea yet - The Aviator Aerial Act! His mechanical marvel was nearly ready - a contraption with colorful carcening carts and spinning seats that whirled riders into the treetops!

But on the eve of opening festivities, disaster struck. Edmund's craft crackled and crumbled, cog work crushed beyond quick repair. "My crowning carnival creation, canceled!" cried the crestfallen creator.

Just then, through the weeping willows came wandering a familiar face with fortuitous offers - the fortune-telling fox Finnegan, friend to all forest folk! "Fear not, my fellow, let me help hatch a hastily hatched new plan to please your patrons come morn!"

They put puzzling pates together and hatched a hilarious hybrid - how about harnessing Whimsical Wood's mischievous moonbeam monkeys as mirthful midway managers? "Fetch them forthwith, fetch enough bananas, and let their antics enchant!"

Come carnival commencement, crowds cascaded into the clearing to find frivolous furry friends flitting from floor to flying trapeze! Their frenetic frolicking kept folks in fits of fun and fascination.

After, attendees were invited into Edmund's Exposition Experience - an emporium of eccentric exhibitions. Mystical menageries, marvelous machinery, and more mysteries amazed all who entered.

In a fabulous finale, Finnegan astounded with illusions too incredible! He conjured creatures from the chaos and called forth a color-changing chameleon, a dancing dragon, and a shrieking sugar glider that sent observers into hysterics!

At dusk, the delighted dignitaries declared this jubilation the jolliest jungle jamboree yet. Thanks to teamwork, troubles were transformed into triumphs sure to be told for years in the whimsical wood!

Title: "Harvesting Memories: Tales from Maple Manor Retirement Home"

Albert sighed as he gazed out the window of Maple Manor Retirement Home. At 78 years old, his mind often wandered to fond recollections of times past on the family farm.

He remembered warm summer days spent roaming the rolling green hills with his siblings - Jane, Sarah, and Henry. They'd spend hours climbing apple trees, splashing in the creek, or having picnic lunches under a towering oak.

Those were simpler times before tractors when chores were done by hand. Albert would rise at dawn to fetch eggs and milk the cows by lantern light. He missed the earthy smells of the barn and the feel of soft fur between his calloused fingers.

As a teenager, Albert took over most of the farm work from his aging father. He worked from sunup til sundown, plowing the fields, baling hay, or repairing fences. Exhausted but content, Albert felt a deep pride in keeping his family's rural heritage alive.

In the evenings, neighbors would gather at the Wilson's for contra dancing under the stars. Albert smiled, recalling Jane's flowery sundresses and strawberry-blonde curls bouncing as she spun across the grass. On quiet nights, he and Jane would stroll hand-in-hand down Lovers Lane.

In 1950, Albert wed sweet Jane in a charming countryside ceremony. They lived happily in a cozy farmhouse, raising three kids - Luke, Molly, and Emma - amid rolling pastures and orchards. In the fall, the family would roast chestnuts on an open fire and press cider from their bountiful apple crop.

But in the 1960s, properties were bought up to make way for construction. As highways stretched across once serene scenery, Albert knew their idyllic way of life was fading. One by one, neighbors sold off, and the family was forced to move to town. Albert retired from carpentry but still missed wide-open skies.

Now at Maple Manor, nostalgia filled Albert's heart for days gone by. But he took comfort knowing farm life lived on in cherished memoirs he shared with friends, like Tom the mailman and Mildred from church. Though times change, memories have the power to reconnect us to the beauty in life's simpler pleasures. And for that, Albert was grateful.

Title: "Tea Time Tales: A Journey through Memories at Maple Manor Retirement Home"

It was a sunny Thursday afternoon at the cozy Maple Manor Retirement Home. In the common room, several residents had gathered for their regular afternoon activity - high tea and conversation with close friends.

Mildred was busy laying out a spectacular spread on her floral tea tablecloth. There were crustless sandwiches with the crusts cut off, homemade scones with lemon curd and clotted cream, and an elegant three-tiered serving stand packed with baked goods.

"I made your favorite cranberry white chocolate cookies, Bernice," said Mildred with a warm smile. Bernice beamed, patting her friend's arm affectionately. Soon the teapot whistled, and Mildred began pouring steaming cups of Earl Grey.

Other residents ambled over, drawn by the enticing aromas. Albert arrived with a tour book of the British Isles in hand. "Thought we could plan some dream vacations while we chat," he suggested cheerfully. Nearby, Tom regaled the group with tales from his newspaper delivery route that morning.

As sugar cubes dissolved and conversations flowed freely, a sense of calm and community filled the air. Mildred reminisced about afternoons spent decorating tiny sandwiches for her mother's social gatherings in the 1950s. Bernice recalled charming English country inns she'd stayed in as a young bride in the 1960s.

Albert pointed out places of interest in Scotland with stories of his grandparents who'd emigrated there in the early 1900s. Tom flipped through his stack of mail showing postcards of European landmarks he hoped to see before he crossed over. Laughter and dreams lifted the friendly group's spirits.

Too soon, the refreshments dwindled. But the magic of tea time lingered on in memories happily shared between fellow travelers down life's journey. Though years and experiences differed greatly, moments like these proved an ageless pleasure - the comfort of companionship over a good cup of tea. It was for this that the residents of Maple Manor were deeply grateful.

Title: "Wheels of Love: A Second Chance at Happiness"

John sighed as he maneuvered his large motorhome through the entrance of Sunny Palms RV Resort. At 65, he never thought he'd be living full-time in an RV, but after his wife passed away last year he couldn't bear to stay in the house they had shared for 40 years.

"Looks like there's a spot open right up front," John said to his dog Hank, who was riding shotgun. John was grateful he had Hank to keep him company in his nomadic lifestyle. As John parked the RV and climbed out, he took a look around at his new residence.

Spread out before him were rows and rows of RVs and campers, with a pool, clubhouse, and other amenities in the center. Palms trees and tropical plants dotted the resort, giving it a warm, relaxing feel. John saw several other residents milling about and hoped he could make some new friends.

Over in site 42, Donna was just finishing her morning coffee on the small porch of her camper. Like John, she found herself living on the road after her husband passed, 3 years ago. Donna loved the freedom of RV life but would be lying if she said she didn't get lonely sometimes.

That's when she noticed the large motorhome pull up across the way. A handsome silver-haired man climbed out and looked around, with a cute little dog by his side. Donna couldn't help smiling, thinking it would be nice to have a neighbor to chat with. Maybe this new man could help cure her loneliness.

A little later, John decided to take Hank for a walk around the resort. As they passed Donna's site, Hank started barking and pulling towards her camper. "Hank, behave!" John scolded. Just then Donna came out.

"Sorry about that, he doesn't usually pull like that," John apologized.

"Oh, it's no trouble, I think he just wants to say hi!" Donna replied with a warm smile. She bent down to pet Hank as the two residents broke the ice, chatting for a while and finding they had a lot in common. Perhaps the RV Resort held more than fun in the sun - it held the promise of new beginnings.

Over the next few weeks, a romance began to blossom between John and Donna as they took their walks together each morning. One sunny Saturday they decided to make a day of it and explore the nearby town. They had lunch at a charming little cafe and browsed the shops, laughing and talking like they were old friends.

On the way back to the resort, John pulled over near a scenic overlook. "Donna, I know we haven't known each other that long but these past few weeks with you have been some of the happiest of my life since Ellen passed," John said, taking her hand. "I care deeply for you. Would you do me the honor of becoming my partner?"

Donna's eyes filled with tears of joy. "Oh John, nothing would make me happier. You've helped fill the hole in my heart left by Bob." She leaned in, and they shared a tender kiss, the start of what they hoped would be a beautiful future together.

From that day on, John and Donna were inseparable, joined at the hip wherever they went around the resort. The other residents couldn't help but smile at the loving couple. One elderly woman remarked to her husband "It gives me hope that there can be happiness and romance even at our age, if you keep your heart open."

Soon fall arrived, and with it the resort's annual RV Blast festival. There was a BBQ cookoff, tug of war, live music, and more. John and Donna helped organize the events, having more fun than anyone. As evening fell, they slowly danced under the stars to an old love song, gazing into each other's eyes and feeling lucky to have found one another.

A year passed in bliss for John and Donna at the RV resort. One night as they stargazed from their campers, John said "You know, I was thinking. We spend almost all our time together anyway, so it seems silly for us to keep two places. Why don't we make it official and combine households?"

Donna beamed. "I think that's a wonderful idea." And so began the work of moving John's motorhome in site to Donna's camper and making them one cozy abode. Their neighbors all pitched in to help, delighted that the cute couple was taking the next step.

Just when they thought things couldn't get better, John and Donna received a surprise. Donna's daughter called to tell them she was expecting - they were going to be grandparents! Overjoyed with the news, they knew what they had to do. It was time to trade four wheels for roots and find a little house near their expanding family.

And so with mixed feelings, John and Donna said goodbye to their resort residence and all the friends they had made there. They would miss the easy lifestyle but were eager to start a new chapter closer to their daughter and the baby. They drove off holding hands, certain the future was bright with their love to guide them. The RV Resort had given them more than they ever imagined - a second chance at happiness and family for their golden years.

Title: "The Retirement Village Caper: Part 1 - A Roll of the Dice"

John Miller had just retired at the age of 65 after a long career as an accountant. While he was looking forward to the leisure of retirement, he was a bit anxious about all the free time he would now have. As an extroverted person, John knew he would get bored sitting at home alone all day. That's why he decided to move into the Sunnydale Retirement Village, hoping to meet new friends and stay active.

On John's first day at the village, he set out to explore his new home and meet his neighbors. He stopped to chat with anyone he passed, introducing himself and asking them questions to learn their stories. That's how John met Marvin, a spry 78-year-old who had lived in Sunnydale for over a decade.

"Welcome to the village! Don't let all the bingo and knitting fool you, things can get pretty wild around here sometimes," Marvin said with a chuckle. John laughed, thinking the old man was pulling his leg. But over the next few months, John discovered that Marvin wasn't joking at all. He soon found himself getting roped into some of the more "unique" activities the residents got up to.

It started small, with a group of seniors deciding to liven up their water aerobics class by trying to sink a bar of soap like a battleship. Before long, they had turned the entire class into an elaborate soap battle game. The instructor was not amused but the residents were having the time of their lives. John had to admit, it was fun to act like a kid again.

Things escalated from there. Marvin let John in on some of the villagers' more daring exploits. For the time Gladys borrowed her grandson's drone and had all the residents take turns trying to knock snacks out of the sky with their walking sticks. Or when Hank hacked into the community center sound system and started blasting the chicken dance music during their monthly board meeting. The pranks and mischief kept everyone on their toes and provided endless entertainment.

But the residents' biggest caper was yet to come. For years, the village board had rejected all proposals for a casino night fundraiser, claiming it promoted gambling. The seniors were tired of boring bingo and card games every Friday. So Marvin hatched an elaborate plan for them to host their underground casino in the basement rec room, complete with blackjack tables, a roulette wheel, and poker.

On the big night, the basement was transformed. With Marvin as the emcee, all the villagers donned their fanciest clothes and got into the spirit, dealing fake chips and cigars added to the atmosphere. Laughter and lively music could be heard echoing through the basement as the residents cut loose far into the night. That was until the village director showed up uninvited...

Title: "An Unexpected Knitting Adventure"

John was feeling bored and unfulfilled in his daily routine. He worked long hours at a desk job he didn't find very interesting, then came home every night just wanting to collapse on the couch. His friends were all getting married and having kids, while he still felt stuck in the same place.

One Saturday while browsing online, an ad popped up suggesting knitting as a new relaxing hobby. John laughed out loud at the idea, thinking it was something only little old ladies did. But after a few minutes of scrolling, his curiosity got the better of him. The patterns and colors of the yarn looked strangely appealing.

On a whim, John decided to give it a try. He drove to the craft store and nervously wandered the aisles, feeling very out of place among all the knitting needles, crochet hooks, and piles of yarn. A kind employee noticed his lost expression and took pity on him. "First time?" she asked with a smile. John admitted the truth, and she helped him pick out some basic supplies to get started.

Sitting at home that night, John fumbled with the needles and yarn, having no idea what he was doing. His first few attempts at casting on came out in a big tangled mess. He was ready to give up when he spotted a beginner tutorial video on YouTube. Slowly following the steps, he managed to get the yarn neatly arranged on the needles. His first knit stitch was clumsy but it worked!

Hooked by the satisfaction of completing that first stitch, John kept practicing. Row by row, his tension evened out, and the speed increased. After a few late nights in front of the television, his initial swatch had grown into a small scarf. John was shocked by his progress and growing enjoyment of the craft.

Word spread among his friends about John's new hobby. "Aren't you a little too manly for knitting?" his buddy Todd joked. But soon enough, Todd's girlfriend Lisa was begging John to make her a scarf for Christmas. Seeing how much pride John took in his growing knitting skills, even Todd had to admit it looked relaxing and creative.

At the next craft store visit, John noticed a flyer advertising a knitting club meeting that week. He shrugged and decided to check it out, curious to meet others who shared his hobby. Much to his surprise, the group wasn't just little old ladies like he expected - there were people of all ages and backgrounds taking part.

John instantly bonded with a group of guys closer to his age who were also relatively new to knitting. Their numbers were growing as the stigma faded. Over crochet hooks and wine, deep conversations flowed as naturally as the stitches. John found himself looking forward to the weekly gatherings, enjoying both the company and creative outlet.

Months passed in a blink, and before John knew it winter was approaching again. He had crafted sweater after sweater, scarf after scarf. Not only was his skill level high, but so were his spirits. Knitting brought John a sense of calm, accomplishment, and community he never expected to find. As he wrapped Lisa's Christmas gifts in festive paper, John smiled at how one small impulsive purchase led to such big life changes. An unexpected knitting adventure indeed!

Title: "An Unexpected Friendship"

Jake was having a terrible day. He had just been laid off from his job, gotten into a fight with his wife, and his car had broken down on the side of the highway on his way home. "Can this day get any worse?" he muttered to himself as a loud clap of thunder echoed across the sky. That's when the rain started to pour.

Soaking wet and frustrated, Jake popped the hood of his car to take a look. But he knew nothing about engines so he had no clue what the problem could be. As he stood there contemplating whether to call for a tow truck, another car pulled over behind him - an older sedan with rust spots all over.

A large man in faded coveralls emerged from the driver's side. "Car trouble eh?" he called out over the sound of the pounding rain. Jake nodded glumly. "Mind if I take a look?" the man asked. Jake shrugged, getting any help he could get at this point.

The man spent a few minutes poking around under the hood before declaring "Ah yep, I see the problem. Your alternator belt snapped. But lucky for you I got a spare in the trunk that should do the job." Within a half hour, the man had the new belt installed and Jake's car was up and running again.

"I appreciate you stopping to help," Jake said gratefully. "Most people probably would have just driven on by. Can I give you some money for the part or buy you a beer or something?" The man waved his hand. "Ah don't worry about it. Name's Burt, by the way."

Over the next few months, Jake and Burt kept running into each other - at the local diner, hardware store, and even a baseball game one weekend. And each time they would stop to chat, finding they surprisingly had a lot in common. Burt was recently widowed and lived alone, and Jake's wife Elizabeth worked long hours at the hospital, so they both welcomed the companionship.

Before long, Burt had taken Jake under his wing, teaching him the basics of auto repair in his spare workshop. And on weekends, they would grab a six-pack and watch sporting events together. Elizabeth was hesitant about their friendship at first but soon warmed up to Burt's kind spirit and humor.

One night as they sat around a bonfire at Burt's, roasting hot dogs, Jake couldn't help but marvel at how such an unlikely bond had formed. As if reading his mind, Burt grinned and said, "Funny how life works sometimes ain't it? When one door closes, another one opens, and you never know what you might find on the other side."

Jake raised his beer in agreement, deeply grateful to have found an unexpected friend just when he needed one most. Their friendship was a reminder that even in difficult times, light can be found in unlikely places if you just keep your head up and your heart open.

Title: "A Weekend to Remember"

Jack was excited for the weekend ahead. It had been far too long since he and his college buddies Dave and Matt had gotten together just to hang out, crack open a few beers, and enjoy each other's company. Between jobs, relationships, and other adult responsibilities, finding time to cut loose was becoming more and more difficult.

But this weekend they were making it a priority. They rented a cabin out in the woods, stocked up on all their favorite snacks and drinks, and packed up the car on Friday after work ready to leave the real world behind for a couple of days.

As they drove up the winding road to the cabin, Jack glanced over at Dave, who was passed out in the passenger seat already drooling on himself. "Some things never change I see," Jack laughed while Matt just smiled and shook his head in the backseat. They arrived just as the sun was beginning to set, painting the sky with beautiful shades of orange and pink.

They hauled their bags inside and immediately cracked open the first beers of the weekend. It felt good to kick back and relax. After catching up on everything they had missed in each other's lives lately, they decided to cook burgers on the grill out back as the stars started to shine bright in the dark blanket of sky above the trees.

Over dinner, they reminisced about wild college memories and continued cracking jokes at each other's expense. The beers kept flowing as they sat around the campfire afterward, feeling perfectly content in each other's company. It had been the perfect start to the weekend.

Late into the night, they finally turned in, exhausted but happy. The next morning they woke to the sun pouring in through the windows, still groggy but glad they didn't have anywhere to be. After scarfing down bowls of Fruity Pebbles, they decided to grab their fishing poles and try their luck at the nearby lake.

A few bites here and there kept their spirits high, but they were just enjoying the relaxation of floating in the peaceful water, far from any buzzing electronics or to-do lists. By midday, they decided to pack it in and throw the few small fish they caught on the grill. Nothing is better than the food you catch yourself, right?

After filling their stomachs, Matt suggested they break out a deck of cards for a few hands of poker to pass the afternoon. Jack and Dave laughed knowing Matt had always been awful at bluffing, which made for some highly entertaining games. A few too many beers in and the jokes and jabs at each other were in full force again.

Just when things were heating up around the table, they heard a roar come from the direction of the cabins. They froze, exchanging confused looks, until suddenly a crowd of motorcycle enthusiasts came into view. It turned out there was some big rally happening nearby that weekend they hadn't known about.

Being the friendly drunk lads they were, Jack and the guys waved the group over to join their game. Before they knew it, poker had turned into a raucous party around their cabin with newfound biker buddies. The beers, shots, and tall tales flowed endlessly into the night. They forgot all about the normal cares and worries of daily life, submerged instead in good company and fun times.

By the end of the weekend, tired but satisfied, they packed up the car Sunday evening with smiles on their faces. They knew they would never forget the debauchery they witnessed and were a part of around that poker table. A fun-filled couple of days exactly as planned - a perfect escape and exactly what they all needed to recharge. Looking back, it was a weekend to remember.

Title: "A Twist of Fate: How I Learned to Love Golf"

Jake had never been interested in golf. As an avid soccer player in his younger days, he saw golf as a boring old man's game. But a chance encounter at the driving range was about to change his mind.

It was a hot Saturday afternoon, and Jake's friends had all bailed on their regular pickup soccer game. Annoyed at being stuck inside on such a nice day, he decided to get some fresh air and grab a bag of balls at the driving range down the road.

As he loaded up his bucket, he overheard the group next to him arguing loudly. "Carl, you've got to change your grip if you ever want to hit the ball straight," one man said sternly. His friend Carl mumbled something unintelligible and stubbornly gripped the club the same way.

Jake chuckled to himself, amused by the spectacle. But his humor quickly turned to shock as Carl took a massive swing, and the club went flying out of his hands, spinning end over end like a boomerang. Time seemed to slow down as Jake watched it sail right at him. He tried to duck but felt a sharp crack on the side of his head before everything went black.

When Jake woke up, he was lying in a hospital bed with a bright white bandage wrapped around his head. A kindly nurse explained that Carl's errant club had given him a concussion but luckily no serious damage. Feeling groggy, Jake wondered how he would explain this golfing accident to his friends who knew his dislike for the sport.

After being released, Jake decided to return to the range a few days later, partly out of curiosity but mostly to confront Carl and demand an explanation. But when he got there, Carl approached him with a hangdog expression, clearly worried about the legal repercussions. "I am so sorry about what happened, I want to make it up to you," Carl said. "Please, let me give you some lessons - I've been playing for 30 years, it's the least I can do."

Figuring it was better than sulking at home, Jake begrudgingly accepted Carl's offer. At first, he was awkward, constantly shanking balls into the surrounding trees or dribbling them along the ground. But Carl was a patient teacher, adjusting Jake's stance and swing with gentle prodding. Slowly but surely, Jake started to hit the ball more solidly and go longer distances.

By the end of the lesson, Jake was enjoying the satisfying crack of hitting the center of the clubface. A feeling of calm had washed over him, replacing his usual stress and worries. Carl smiled. "See, there's more to golf than most people realize. It's about focus and feeling as much as strength. Glad you're starting to see that."

From that day on, Jake began spending more and more days at the driving range, his bag of clubs growing heavier with new equipment. His friends were shocked by the transformation but started joining him on the course for casual weekend rounds. Jake even signed up for a local beginner's league, where he met Carol, a single mom who also loved the sport.

Who would have thought that getting beaned in the head by a flying golf club would change his life so dramatically? Jake was grateful for his twist of fate and all the joy golf had brought into his life since. It just goes to show you never know what adventure is around the corner.

Title: "A Day at the Bakery"

John woke up excited for his first day of work at his new job. After being unemployed for months, he was happy to finally land a position at the bakery down the street. He threw on his uniform, a classic white t-shirt and jeans, and headed out the door.

When John arrived, the smell of freshly baked bread immediately lifted his spirit. "Mmm, something smells good in here," he said as he walked through the door. His boss Sally greeted him with a warm smile. "Great to have you, John. We open in 10 minutes, so let me show you the ropes."

Sally showed John around the small bakery, introducing him to the ovens, mixers, racks of bread, and cases filled with sweets. "I'll be baking in the back, so you'll be upfront helping customers. Think you can handle the register?" John nodded confidently. How hard could it be?

The first customer walked in just as they opened. "Welcome to the bakery! What can I get for you?" John asked cheerfully. The man looked over the displays intently. After several long minutes, he finally said, "I'll take one of those croissants, please." John proudly bagged up the pastry and accepted the customer's payment. One down, who knows how many more to go!

As the morning went on, John got more comfortable with the routines. He smiled and greeted everyone who walked through the door. By lunchtime, the case was looking bare. That's when Sally poked her head out of the back. "Hey John, we're almost out of a few things. Do you think you can lend me a hand back here for a bit?"

John nervously replied, "Sure, I'll do my best!" He walked to the back and was greeted by the chaotic but organized mess that was a commercial bakery kitchen. Flour coated every surface. Doughs were rising all over, and mixing bowls filled with batters waited to become loaf pans of delicious bread. "Alright, let's get you started kneading some dough," Sally instructed.

As John worked the dough, it became messier but also more satisfying. The rhythmic motion was somehow soothing. Sally showed him techniques to stretch and fold it just right. Before he knew it, he had a smooth, elastic ball ready for rising. "Great work!" Sally exclaimed. She was genuinely impressed with how fast he picked it up.

Thanks to John's help, they were fully stocked again in no time. The rest of the day flew by in a blur of customers, baking, and friendly chatting. At the end of his shift, John's feet hurt, but his heart was full. As he looked around at the nearly empty cases, he felt proud to have contributed to all those smiling customers. "Well John, what do you think? Want to come back tomorrow?" Sally asked sincerely.

John laughed and replied, "Are you kidding?! I loved every messy minute of it. I'll see you bright and early." With that, he said his goodbyes and headed home, already looking forward to the next day. Who knew that a little humble bakery could fill him with such joy? John sure was glad he took a chance on this new career. It seemed he had found exactly where he was meant to be.

Title: "An Interesting Conversation over Coffee"

John was having a busy day at the office and was looking forward to taking a coffee break. As he sat down at the small cafe nearby with his latte, he noticed a woman sitting alone reading a book. She seemed engrossed in her reading and had a gentle smile on her face.

Not wanting to disturb her, John started sipping his coffee and checking emails on his phone. A few minutes later, the woman put her book down and sighed. As if on cue, her coffee cup was empty too. She looked around like she was contemplating getting a refill.

On an impulse, John said to her, "Looks like we're both due for a refill. Can I get the next one for you?" She looked up, a little surprised but smiled warmly and said, "Why yes, thank you. That's very kind of you."

John went to the counter and got them both a refill. As he brought it over, he said, "I hope you don't mind me interrupting your reading. It just looked like the perfect time for a coffee break." She laughed lightly and said, "Not at all, the book had me hooked but the break is welcome. I'm Claire by the way." "Nice to meet you Claire, I'm John," he said as he extended his hand.

They spent the next half an hour chatting casually. Claire told him about being an engineer and working on designing sustainable buildings. John was fascinated by her passion for her work and her ideas. She, in turn, was interested to learn about his job in financial advising. Before they knew it, they had finished two more refills each while lost in their discussion.

As they both looked at their empty cups again, Claire said, "Well, I think it's time to get back to work now, but I've enjoyed our conversation. It's not every day you meet someone as interesting to talk to over coffee." John replied, "Same here, the time just flew by. Would you like to do this again sometime, maybe over dinner?"

Claire smiled, a little shyly this time, "I'd love to. How about this weekend?" They exchanged numbers, and John walked back to the office with a spring in his step. As strange as it seemed, one casual conversation over coffee had led to what he hoped was the beginning of something special.

Title: "An Unexpected Connection"

John was rushing to work like he did every morning, barely taking time to enjoy his coffee in the car. As he sped down the highway, he noticed the traffic starting to slow up ahead. "Ugh, not now, I'm going to be late," he said to himself impatiently.

When he got closer, he could see an accident had just occurred; a car had swerved off the road and crashed into the trees. John begrudgingly stopped his car and got out, figuring he should at least see if anyone needed help. As he approached the wrecked vehicle, he saw a woman still sitting in the driver's seat, shaking with fear.

"Ma'am, are you alright? Are you injured?" John asked with concern. The woman looked up with tears in her eyes. "I think so, I'm just in shock. It all happened so fast," she replied. John called 911 and reported the accident while he waited with the woman to calm her nerves. After what seemed like forever, the ambulance and police arrived to take over.

As John began to walk back to his car, he heard a soft voice behind him, "Thank you for stopping to help me; I appreciate you staying until the emergency crews got here." He turned to see the woman now standing, a blanket wrapped around her shoulders. "You're very welcome. I'm just glad you aren't seriously hurt. What's your name?" John asked. "Samantha," she replied with a small smile.

Over the next few weeks, John couldn't get Samantha out of his mind. There was something about her soothing voice and kind eyes that he found intriguing. After mustering up the courage, he decided to go to the local coffee shop in hopes of running into her again. Lo and behold, after about 15 minutes of casually sipping his coffee by the window, Samantha walked through the door.

Thrilled by the coincidence, John wasted no time in going up and introducing himself. They sat and talked for hours, realizing they had much more in common than just the random accident that brought them together initially. An undeniable spark was ignited between them from that chance meeting.

Before they knew it, a friendship had blossomed into something more. John was happier than he'd been in a long time having Samantha by his side. They made each other laugh while also providing the comfort and support each needed. The feelings they developed for each other felt so natural and right.

One year later, on their anniversary of meeting, John planned a romantic picnic in the park near where they first reunited. As they sat gazing up at the stars after dinner, John took Samantha's hands in his. "From the moment I saw you shaking and scared in your car that day, I knew there was something special about you. You've brought so much joy into my life, and I can't imagine it without you. Will you make me the luckiest man and marry me?" he asked nervously.

Through happy tears, Samantha replied, "Yes, yes, of course, I'll marry you!". They sealed their engagement with a long loving kiss, grateful that fate led this unexpected connection to blossom into true love.

Title: "The Bonds that Transcend Time"

The leaves were just starting to change color in the small rural town of Oakdale. John Davidson sat on his front porch enjoying a cup of coffee and the tranquility of the Saturday morning. As he gazed out at the large oak trees dotted across his property, his mind wandered to thoughts of his family and friends.

It had been nearly 10 years since John and his wife Mary had moved to Oakdale after retiring from their jobs in the city. They wanted to slow down and spend more quiet time together in a place less hectic than the life they had become accustomed to. Oakdale provided just what they were searching for. Over the years, they had come to know and cherish the tight-knit community and the bonds they had formed with their neighbors. But John was feeling restless lately and thought it might be nice to reconnect with old friends from years past.

As John sipped his coffee, a moving van rolled down the street, catching his attention. He watched with curiosity as boxes and furniture were carefully offloaded from the large vehicle. A middle-aged couple supervised the crew, directing where to place items in the small ranch-style home at the end of the block. Once everything was inside, the movers packed up and drove away, leaving the couple alone on their new porch.

John finished his coffee and headed over to introduce himself and welcome the new neighbors. As he approached, the woman spotted him and waved. "Good morning! I'm Susan, and this is my husband Mark. We just moved here from the city, glad to meet someone friendly already." John smiled and replied, "Welcome to Oakdale! I'm John, I live just down the street. Always happy to meet new folks settling in around here. Let me know if you need any help unpacking or have any questions about the area."

Over the next few hours, John helped Mark and Susan unpack boxes and get settled into their new home. As they worked, the three began sharing stories of their lives and experiences. John spoke fondly of retiring to Oakdale with his wife and the pleasures of small-town living. Mark talked about his career in finance that had them moving often for work. But Susan seemed most excited to finally put down roots after years of relocating.

As they emptied the last box, John was shocked to realize he knew Susan from long ago. "Susan Wilson...is that you? It must be over 30 years, but I'd recognize that smile anywhere! We went to high school together, if I'm not mistaken." Susan examined John's face more closely, and her eyes lit up. "Well, I'll be, John Davidson! I never thought I'd run into a familiar face out here. How have you been all these years?"

The two old friends spent the rest of the afternoon reminiscing and catching up on the decades that passed since they last saw each other. John was overjoyed to have reconnected with a friend from his youth in such a serendipitous way.

In the following weeks, John introduced Susan and Mark to Mary and the rest of their friends in Oakdale. It was like the couple had always been a part of the close community. On weekends they would have cookouts and exchange stories while the children played. Susan and John continued to bond over memories of high school and reminisce about changes in their hometown over the decades. Their lives had taken different paths since the bond of friendship that started so long ago proved to transcend time and distance. Susan and Mark found the roots and sense of belonging they had searched for, and John's longing for nostalgia was fulfilled in the most heartwarming of ways. The strength of family and friendship proved eternal in the small town of Oakdale.

Title: "Connections"

The rush hour traffic moved at a crawl as Jack stared impatiently at the clock. His flight was boarding in 30 minutes and the airport was still 20 miles away. "Please let me make this flight," he muttered to no one in particular.

Just then, his phone rang with an unknown number. "Hello?" he answered cautiously. "Hi, is this Jack Smith?" said a cheerful voice on the other end. "Yes, this is Jack." "Great! This is Angelica from Airport Connections. I'm calling because it looks like you might miss your flight if you sit in this traffic much longer. We're a service that provides alternative transportation to the airport in situations just like this. How soon do you need to be at the airport?"

Jack checked the boarding time again. "In about 25 minutes," he replied, a hint of panic in his voice. "Okay, don't worry," Angelica assured him calmly. "I'm sending a driver to your location right now. What's the best place for him to find you?" Jack gave her the cross streets of where he was stuck. "Alright, he'll be there in 5 minutes. Just look for a blue sedan. You're gonna make your flight, I promise!"

Sure enough, right on time a blue sedan pulled up next to Jack's car. The driver climbed out and introduced himself as Miguel. "Follow me, I'll get you to the airport fast but safe," Miguel said with a smile. Jack jumped out, throwing a grateful look over his shoulder as Miguel guided him expertly through side streets and shortcuts Jack never would have thought of.

In what seemed like no time at all, they were whipping into the airport arrivals lane. Miguel screeched to a halt right at the entrance. "Go, you've got 15 minutes before boarding ends!" Jack threw some cash at Miguel and jumped out, shouting "Thank you!" over his shoulder as he sprinted into the terminal.

He dashed up to the counter, chest heaving, as the agent was just calling the final boarding call. "I'm here...flight to Chicago...please..." he panted. The agent scanned his ID and boarding pass. "Just made it sir, have a good flight!"

As Jack collapsed into his seat, breathing a sigh of relief, he pulled out his phone to send Angelica a message. But then he had another idea. He pulled up the Airport Connections website and left a glowing review, making sure to call out Miguel and Angelica by name for going above and beyond.

A few days later, as Miguel was driving another frantic passenger to the airport, he got a notification on his phone. It was a message from the company: "Wow, thanks to your amazing work, we just got an endorsement that's helping business take off. Keep up the great service!" Miguel smiled, feeling glad to have played a small role in helping people's important travels stay on track. It was nice to end a day knowing he had Connections someone to where they urgently needed to be.

Title: "A Perfect Hike...Almost"

Jim sighed as he looked out the window at the rain pouring down. He had been looking forward to this weekend for months. It was supposed to be the annual guys' hiking trip. Every year, he and his friends would pack up for two days and head into the woods for some camping, hiking, fishing, and lots of beers by the campfire.

But Mother Nature had other plans. The weather report was calling for rain all weekend long. Jim was just about to send the group a text canceling the trip when his phone buzzed with a message from his friend Dave.

"Rain or shine boys, we're still going! I've got an idea that will make this the best trip ever. Pack your gear and I'll fill you in when you get here."

Against his better judgment, Jim started throwing his backpack and gear into the car. What could Dave possibly have up his sleeve to make a rainy weekend in the woods fun?

A few hours later, Jim pulled up to Dave's house where the rest of the guys were already waiting. "Alright Dave, what's this grand master plan of yours?" Jim asked.

Dave just grinned that grin that usually meant he was up to no good. "Gentlemen, we are no longer taking a regular hiking trip. This weekend, we are embarking on the ultimate adventure - glamping!"

The guys all looked at each other, confused. "Glamping?" Asked Steve "Isn't that where people pay hundreds to sleep in tents with luxurious bedding and amenities?"

"Exactly!" Said Dave "I've got it all taken care of. Follow me and prepare to have your minds blown."

Dave led them around back to what looked like a full-size cabin in the backyard. "Tada!" He yelled, throwing the door open.

Inside, it was better than any luxury hotel suite. There was a full kitchen, a huge flat-screen TV, plush couches, and even a hot tub on the back deck.

"Dave, how in the world..." Jim stammered.

"My cousin owns a glamping resort and was looking for a place to store and demo some of their high-end camping packages over the winter. I told him we'd be the perfect guinea pigs. We've got this whole cabin, plus hot tubs, a sauna, and all the food and drinks you could dream of, completely free for the weekend!"

The guys all cheered, amazed at Dave's brilliance. This trip was going to be perfect after all.

Over the next two days, they feasted on gourmet meals cooked in the kitchen, stayed warm and toasty by the indoor fireplace playing games and telling stories, and relaxed in the hot tub under the stars, beers in hand. It was everything a guy's weekend in the woods could ask for without ever having to worry about the rain.

On the last morning, they decided to do one last hike before packing up and heading home. The rain had finally stopped overnight so the trails would be muddy but hikeable. An hour into the lush forest path, the skies opened up again.

Within minutes, they were soaked to the bone. Visibility was low in the heavy rainfall. Then, without warning, Jim slipped on the slick mud and tumbled down a steep embankment, coming to rest at the bottom in a sizable mud puddle.

The guys rushed over to check on him, hoping he wasn't hurt. To their relief, Jim popped up from the bog, covered from head to toe in thick, brown sludge but otherwise unharmed.

He took one look at his friends' shocked faces and couldn't help but laugh. Soon, they were all howling with laughter at the absurd situation they found themselves in.

Two days of pure luxury and relaxation came to a perfectly fitting end, with five best friends reunited in the mud and rain, just like the old days. Some things, like brotherhood and making memories, are worth getting a little dirty for. As they hiked back to start the journey home, Jim couldn't help but think this would go down as their most perfect hike, almost."

Title: "Balancing Act: The Trials and Triumphs of a Uni Student"

Jenna was exhausted as she walked across her university campus after her last class of the day. As a third-year student majoring in psychology, she had a very full course load and was always pushing herself to do better. She was hoping to graduate with honors and get into a top graduate program, which meant she had to get top marks.

While Jenna found her classes interesting, the workload was starting to take its toll. On top of going to classes, she spent all her free time studying in the library or doing assignments in her tiny dorm room. She was also working a part-time job on the weekends to help pay for living expenses since student loans only covered so much. By the end of each week, she was running on empty.

As she walked, Jenna started daydreaming about all the things she wished she had time for, like going out with friends, joining campus clubs, and going on dates. Her social life had disappeared over the last couple of years, and she was starting to feel lonely. She knew that taking a break was important for her mental health and enjoyment of life, but it was so hard to pry herself away from her books.

Lost in thought, Jenna accidentally walked straight into another student who was rushing across the path. "Oh gosh, I'm so sorry!" she exclaimed, looking up. It was Mike, a handsome guy from her statistics class who she had a bit of a crush on. He laughed it off good-naturedly. "No problem! I should have been watching where I was going too. Long day?" he asked sympathetically.

Jenna sighed. "The longest. I'm exhausted but still have three more chapters to read before tomorrow." Mike nodded understandingly. "I know what that's like. Listen, a bunch of us are getting together at the campus pub in a bit for some much-needed unwinding. Why don't you come to join us? I promise we won't keep you too late." Jenna hesitated, torn between wanting to go and also feeling like she had too much work. Mike seemed to sense her indecision. "One hour, that's all. Then you can go home and study to your heart's content. What do you say?"

Against her better judgment, Jenna agreed. One hour surely wouldn't hurt, right? She ended up having such a great time laughing and joking with Mike and his friends that she quite forgot about her schoolwork for a while. They talked about everything from their classes to current events to their summer plans. Jenna realized how much she needed this social interaction and stress relief.

As the last call was announced, Mike walked Jenna back to her dorm. "Thanks for coming out tonight. I'm glad I ran into you, literally," he said with a smile. Jenna smiled back shyly. "Me too. And thanks for inviting me, I needed the break." Impulsively, Mike leaned in and kissed her softly. "How about we do this again sometime, but make it a date?" he asked. Jenna beamed. "I'd like that."

Waving goodbye to Mike, Jenna went inside feeling happier than she had in ages. She realized that while school was important, it wasn't everything. Making time for relationships and fun was just as vital for her health and happiness. From then on, Jenna committed to maintaining a better work-life balance, studying hard but also making sure to go out with friends regularly to recharge. She even started dating Mike, who proved to be very supportive of her dreams.

Through organization, self-care, and keeping perspective on what truly mattered to her, Jenna successfully finished her degree with honors while also enjoying her university experience to the fullest. She proved that it was possible to have the best of both worlds through balance and prioritizing well-being. Jenna's time at university, with all its trials and triumphs, had given her skills and relationships that would last a lifetime.

Title: "The Wedding Planners: An Unexpected Pairing"

Jenny sighed as she looked through photos of yet another bride who was having a complete meltdown on her Pinterest-perfect wedding day. As one of the top wedding planners in the city, it was Jenny's job to swoop in during these disasters and save the day. She loved the challenge but sometimes the stress got to her.

As she scrolled through her emails, one caught her eye from an unfamiliar sender named Steve. "Need an emergency wedding planner - groomsmen all have food poisoning!" it read. Jenny chuckled and wondered what kind of trouble his wedding was in. She called the number, and Steve answered frantically. "Thank god you called back! Half my party is ill, and my planner just quit - please tell me you can help!"

After getting the details, Jenny hopped in her car and headed to the venue. When she arrived, she found Steve running around like a madman, still in his suit. She introduced herself and took charge of the situation immediately. "Alright, let's assess what we have to work with here." She got the caterer on the phone to rearrange the meals and told some of the unaffected groomsmen to help set up extra tables outside for more guests.

Through creative problem-solving and calm leadership, Jenny got the wedding back on track just in time. As the reception began, an impressed Steve came to thank her. "I don't know what we would have done without you. How can I ever repay you?" he asked. Jenny laughed. "Just doing my job! I'm glad I could help salvage your special day."

Over the next few months, Steve and Jenny stayed in touch as friends. Jenny discovered that under his frenzied best-man exterior, Steve was a thoughtful guy with a great sense of humor. They had amazing chemistry when hanging out. Soon they started dating, much to Jenny's surprise, since wedding planners aren't supposed to fraternize with clients!

One year later, Jenny was happy but busy preparing for a huge celebrity wedding. She got a call from her assistant that Steve was at her office with an urgent matter. When she walked out, Steve was down on one knee holding an open ring box. "Jenny, will you do me the honor of becoming my wife?" he asked, nerves evident in his shaking voice.

Jenny was stunned, both by the proposal and realizing her true feelings for Steve. Though the timing wasn't ideal, she said yes immediately, throwing her arms around him joyfully. They planned a small, intimate ceremony for a few months later so Jenny could finish her work commitments.

On their wedding day, Jenny laughed thinking of how they met - her saving Steve's disastrous wedding. Who would have thought that event would lead them to find love with each other? Thanks to a crazy sequence of events, Jenny discovered that wedding planning wasn't just her career but also her happy ending. Their reception was filled with laughter, tears, and plenty of inside jokes about food-poisoning groomsmen. It truly was the best day ever.

Title: "The Final Countdown: Surviving Exam Season"

Adam anxiously paced the halls of his high school, books in hand. It was the night before his first major exam, and he was unprepared. How did he let things get to this point? Over the past few months, he had been so busy with sports, work, and his social life that studying fell by the wayside. Now he was facing the consequences.

As he walked, fretting about the Disastrous Exam Disaster (that's what he was calling it in his head), Adam crashed right into his friend Sarah. "Oof, watch it!" she exclaimed. Then seeing the panicked look on his face, she asked, "Exam crazies got you too, huh?" Adam nodded miserably.

Sarah smiled sympathetically. "I know things look bad now, but it's not over yet. Come to the library with me; I'll help you cram." Two boring but productive hours later found Adam's head swimming with dates, facts, and formulas. It wasn't a full mastery of the material, but it was a start.

That night he barely slept, tossing and turning with visions of failing grades. But he got through the exam somehow, thanks to Sarah's last-minute save. After turning in his paper, Adam collapsed onto a nearby bench in relief. "Well, it's out of my hands now," he sighed to Sarah. She patted his back. "You did your best. Now on to the next one!"

And so began their exam season ritual - cramming madly in the library until closing, chugging unhealthy amounts of coffee, and pulling multiple all-nighters. Adam slowly started getting the hang of managing his time better. He wasn't acing everything, but his grades were trending up, which was enough for now.

During one of their late-night study sessions, Sarah surprised Adam by confessing she developed feelings for him over these high-stress weeks of bonding. He realized with a start that he felt the same way. After they finished their last finals, Adam asked Sarah on a celebratory date.

Years later at their wedding, Adam reminisced in his toast about how managing that make-or-break exam period was a practice run for handling the stresses of adult life and relationships. He was grateful Sarah had been there to save him, both academically and romantically. Who would have thought surviving the Exam Disaster would lead him to find his future wife and best friend? Their marriage was a testament to growing together through challenging times with patience, humor, and support.

Title: "Teacher's Pet Project"

Mr. Johnson was tired. He had been teaching high school science for over 30 years and felt like he had seen it all. The fights in the halls, the failed experiments that somehow always caused a mess, and of course the ever-present sea of disinterested faces that made up his classes. It was going to be a long year.

On the first day of classes, Mr. Johnson went through the usual introductions and lab safety spiel. As he looked out at the sea of faces, one stood out to him - a bright-eyed kid in the front row named Timmy. While the other students looked half-asleep already, Timmy sat at attention, soaking up every word. "Well, at least I'll have one engaged student this year," Mr. Johnson thought to himself.

Over the coming weeks, Timmy proved to be Mr. Johnson's star pupil. He aced every test, asked thoughtful questions, and seemed genuinely excited about science. While the rest of the class struggled to stay awake, Timmy was a breath of fresh air. But Mr. Johnson started to notice that Timmy always came to school alone and sat by himself at lunch. He decided he needed to find out more.

The next day, Mr. Johnson asked Timmy to stay after class. "Timmy, I've been impressed with your work so far. You have a science talent. But I've noticed you always seem to be by yourself. Is everything okay?" At first, Timmy was shy, but he eventually opened up to Mr. Johnson, telling him about his divorced parents, lack of friends, and feeling like an outsider. Mr. Johnson's heart broke for the kind but lonely boy. He wanted to help.

That's when Mr. Johnson came up with an idea - he would start a weekly after-school science club and make Timmy his teacher's pet, assisting with experiments and mentoring other students. At first, it was just the two of them, but word spread, and soon the club grew to a dozen students. For the first time, Timmy had friends who shared his passion. Under Mr. Johnson's guidance, Timmy came out of his shell.

Over the year, Timmy helped lead experiments, tutored struggling students, and found his place. On the last day of school, the science club threw Mr. Johnson a surprise retirement party, complete with a scrapbook of photos and letters of gratitude from all the students whose lives he had impacted - including Timmy, who had blossomed from a shy boy into a confident young man ready to take on the world, thanks to one teacher who cared enough to give him a chance. As Mr. Johnson looked out at the group of happy kids, he didn't feel tired anymore - he felt a deep sense of pride and accomplishment. It had been his best year of teaching ever.

Title: "The Last Day and Memories That Will Last"

Jake woke up and sighed as he looked at the calendar. It was his last day at the marketing firm he had worked at for the past 10 years. So much had changed over that time. When he first started, the company was much smaller. They worked out of a run-down office building with only 10 other employees. Now they had grown exponentially and employed over 100 people across three floors in a high-rise downtown.

As he got ready, Jake couldn't help but reminisce on all the memories he had made with his coworkers over the past decade. There was Sarah from accounting whom he had become close friends. They would often grab lunch together and gab about their personal lives. She was the first person he told when he and his wife were expecting their first child. Sarah had cried tears of joy for them.

Then there was Tom in sales who always found a way to make everyone laugh with his hilarious antics and Dad jokes. No matter how stressful things got at the office, Tom could brighten the mood. Their annual "ugly Christmas sweater" contests became the stuff of office legend thanks to Tom's outlandish and often outrageous sweater choices.

When Jake arrived at the office, the atmosphere was surprisingly somber for his last day. He expected a big farewell party but instead, it seemed like everyone was going out of their way to make his last few hours as comfortable as possible. Sarah brought him a breakfast sandwich and coffee from his favorite cafe. Tom had filled his desk with balloons and a giant card signed by the whole department.

As Jake made his rounds saying goodbye to everyone individually, the emotions started to hit him. This place had become his second home and these people were his extended family. He had seen coworkers come and go but never imagined this day would come for him.

At lunch, Sarah, Tom, and a few others insisted on taking him out. As they sat around the table swapping stories, Jake was overcome thinking about how much he would miss this. The camaraderie, the inside jokes, even the little annoyances - it had all become a part of his daily routine. These people had been there for all the big moments in his life and he had theirs.

On the walk back, Sarah linked her arm to Jake's and said "You know we're all going to stay in touch. This isn't goodbye, just see you later. And we expect lots of visits from you!" Jake smiled, feeling a bit better knowing this chapter was closing but the friendships would last forever.

As the end of the day neared, Jake started to pack up his desk amidst a steady stream of well-wishers stopping by. He came across an old photo of himself, Sarah, and Tom from the company holiday party years ago. They all looked so young back then. He smiled, remembering how far they had all come both professionally and personally since that photo.

Tom popped in "Alright big guy, it's time. Everything wrapped up here?" Jake nodded, taking one final look around the office that had been his home for a decade. As they walked to the elevator together, Jake felt a tinge of sadness but also gratitude for the wonderful people and memories that would stay with him forever from his time at this company. It wasn't goodbye, it was just 'see you later' and he looked forward to creating new memories with his coworker-turned-friends in the years to come.

Title: "The Crazy Crew"

John woke up to the sound of his alarm blaring at 6 am sharp as it did every weekday morning. He groaned and rolled over, not ready to face another day at the office. But he forced himself out of bed and into the shower to begin getting ready for work.

As he made his coffee and breakfast, he thought about his coworkers that he would be dealing with for the next 8 hours. There was Sheila, the chatty receptionist who always seemed to be gossiping about someone. Bob from accounting took everything way too seriously and had no sense of humor. And Jeff, the intern, who was still learning the ropes but always seemed to be causing some sort of minor disaster around the office.

When John arrived at the office a little after 7 am, he wasn't surprised to find Sheila already at her desk, on the phone with one of her friends. "Oh my god, you'll never believe what Becky was wearing to the company Christmas party last year!" she was saying loudly. John just shook his head and gave her a wave as he walked to his cubicle.

But it was only a few minutes before Sheila came popping over the half wall. "John, did you hear about Linda in marketing? She's been having an affair with the new guy in sales!" John just sighed. "Sheila, it's not even 8 am yet. Can we please save the gossip for later?" Sheila huffed and went back to her desk, no doubt to call someone else with the latest "dirt".

John settled in at his desk and booted up his computer, hoping for a relaxing morning of catching up on emails and reports. But about an hour later, Bob appeared, frantically waving a stack of papers. "John, I think there's been a mistake in the accounting for last quarter. The numbers just aren't adding up. We need to get to the bottom of this right away before the boss finds out!" John tried to calmly explain to Bob that one missed decimal point wasn't the end of the world but Bob just rushed back to his cubicle, muttering about lawsuits.

Just when John was starting to make some progress on his work, there was a bang and a crash from the break room. He sighed and got up to investigate. Sure enough, there was Jeff, covered head to toe in coffee grounds, with the broken coffee maker at his feet. "I'm so sorry!" Jeff said, eyes wide. "I was just trying to refill it and it just...exploded!" John spent the next 20 minutes helping clean up the mess while Jeff apologized profusely.

By the time lunch rolled around, John was ready to pull his hair out. Every time he turned around, one of his crazy coworkers was causing some new havoc. As he walked to the nearby sandwich shop to grab a quick bite, he wondered how he was going to make it through the rest of the day sane.

But when John got back, he noticed something strange. The office was completely quiet. Too quiet. He slowly made his way back to his desk, half expecting to find it on fire or something equally disastrous. But everything seemed normal. He sat down and continued working, waiting for the next explosion to happen.

A few hours passed with nothing but blissful, productive silence. Finally, curiosity got the better of John and he went to investigate what was going on. He found Sheila, Bob, and Jeff all in the conference room, deeply engrossed in a game of Cards Against Humanity. Laughter and good-natured trash talk filled the air. John leaned in the doorway, smiling as he watched his usually chaotic coworkers getting along and simply having fun together. Maybe they weren't so crazy after all. And maybe working with them wasn't so bad, as long as they could find ways to let off steam like this every once in a while. With that thought, John joined in the next hand, happy to be part of the crew.

Title: "The Unlikely Fitness Buddies"

Jerry pulled into the parking lot of the Silver Springs Community Center with reluctance. At 75 years old, the idea of spending time at the gym was not exactly how he wanted to spend his retirement. But his daughter Sally had insisted, saying it would be good for him to get more exercise and social interaction. As Jerry got out of his car, he sighed deeply wondering how he got talked into this.

He made his way into the large gymnasium area where various fitness classes were taking place. Jerry peeked in on a yoga class full of laughing older women in the poses. Too girly for him, he thought and kept walking. Next, he stopped at the spinning class and watched as a group of men and women his age vigorously pedaled their bikes, cheering each other on. No way was Jerry getting on one of those death traps.

Just then, he spotted the weight room in the back corner. Ah ha, this was more his speed. Lifting some dumbbells and getting his arms pumped, now that sounded like a good workout. As Jerry entered the weight room, he was surprised to see it wasn't empty like he hoped. In the far corner, a petite older woman with short grey hair was lifting a set of hand weights with perfect form.

Jerry wandered over to the set of dumbbells along the wall, hoping to go unnoticed. But the woman spotted him. "Good morning!" she said brightly. "My name is Mildred, are you new here?" Caught off guard, Jerry responded "Uh yeah, first time. Name's Jerry." Mildred smiled warmly. "Welcome, Jerry. Can I show you how to use any of the machines?" Jerry scratched his head, embarrassed. "Well, to be honest, I don't know what I'm doing."

"Not a problem!" replied Mildred. "I'm happy to help. Why don't we start with some basic dumbbell exercises to get your muscles warmed up?" Against his better judgment, Jerry found himself agreeing. Over the next 30 minutes, Mildred took Jerry through a full upper-body dumbbell circuit, correcting his form and cheering him on.

To his surprise, Jerry was starting to sweat by the end. And even more surprising, he was having fun following Mildred's lead. Who would have thought lifting weights could be enjoyable? As they finished up, Mildred asked "So same time next week?" Jerry paused, then said "You know what? Sure, I'll be here."

And so an unlikely friendship and fitness partnership were born. Every Tuesday and Thursday found Jerry meeting Mildred in the weight room at 10 am sharp. Under her tutelage, he learned proper lifting techniques to work his whole body. But more than that, they started looking forward to their time to catch up on each other's lives.

Jerry learned that Mildred's husband had passed away the year before, and she was lonely in her big empty house. Meanwhile, Jerry's wife had left him years ago, and his kids lived out of state, so he spent too much time alone as well. They filled a social void for each other. Before long, Jerry and Mildred were meeting for coffee after their workouts to chat for hours, laughing together like old friends.

One day after a particularly tough leg workout, Jerry and Mildred collapsed onto the gym floor, giggling and out of breath. "I can't feel my quads!" chuckled Jerry. Looking over at his friend, he said more seriously "You know Mildred, I'm really glad you approached me that first day. I never thought I'd say this, but I'm having fun getting in shape. And more than that, I've gained a real friend through all this."

Mildred smiled warmly and patted Jerry's hand. "Me too Jerry. I'm glad we're in this together." At that moment, a spark passed between them that had been growing over months of companionship. Hesitantly, Jerry leaned over and kissed Mildred sweetly. To his relief and joy, she kissed him back. Who would have guessed the silver foxes would find more than exercise when they walked into the gym that day? Their children would later joke that they became fitness - and relationship - goals for seniors everywhere.
Title: "Defending the Man Who Got Away"

Jenna sighed as she looked over the case file on her desk for what felt like the hundredth time. As one of the top defense attorneys in town, she was used to difficult clients - but this one felt nearly impossible. Across the folder in bold lettering was the name "Jason Roberts" - her high school sweetheart and the man who got away.

They had dated throughout their senior year of high school and even into their first year of college. Jenna had been head over heels for Jason and thought they would be together forever. But in their sophomore year, Jason started pulling away. He became distant and their fights became more frequent. Eventually, he broke things off, claiming he just wasn't ready for such a serious commitment. The breakup crushed Jenna.

Now, nearly 10 years later, here he was sitting in an interrogation room, being charged with grand theft auto. According to the files, Jason had allegedly stolen his ex-wife's car during a heated argument over their divorce settlement. The DA was pushing for jail time, claiming this was proof of an escalating pattern of violence and control.

Jenna knew she should recuse herself, that defending an ex would be a major conflict of interest. But when Jason pleaded with her on the phone, begging for her help, she couldn't say no. So with a reluctant sigh, she grabbed her briefcase and made her way to the police station.

When she entered the interrogation room, her heart skipped a beat at the sight of Jason. He hadn't changed much over the years - still with those piercing blue eyes and charming smile. But this time, the smile didn't quite reach his eyes. She could see the exhaustion and regret etched on his face.

"Thanks for coming, Jen. I appreciate you taking my case," Jason said softly.

Jenna nodded curtly. "Let's not dwell on old relationships right now. Tell me exactly what happened."

Over the next hour, Jason recounted his side of the story. It was clear things with the ex-wife had become volatile during their divorce. While he admitted to taking the car, he claimed it was out of anger at the moment rather than a pre-meditated plan. Jenna wasn't sure what to believe, torn between her past feelings for Jason and her duty as his attorney.

The day of the trial arrived. Jenna pored over the evidence for every angle she could spin in Jason's favor. However, the DA was persistent, presenting Jason as an abuser who needed to be locked away. During closing statements, Jenna gave it her all, appealing to the judge and jury's humanity. She believed everyone deserved a fair chance at redemption.

To her surprise and relief, the jury found Jason not guilty. As he was released from custody, Jason rushed over to hug Jenna. "Thank you...for everything. I owe you big time," he said gratefully. Jenna smiled, feeling like maybe some old wounds were starting to heal.

In the months that followed, Jason worked hard to get his life back on track. He and Jenna began spending time together as friends, and she was glad to see him transforming into the caring, thoughtful man she once knew. One night over drinks, Jason confessed he never stopped thinking about her all these years. And to Jenna's surprise, she realized her feelings for him remained, buried but not gone.

Sometimes, second chances are what we need to find our way back to where we belong.

Title: "The Prankster Gets Pranked: Revenge is Sweet (But Not as Sweet as Cake)"

Mark had always been the biggest prankster amongst his friends. Birthdays, holidays, random Tuesdays - no occasion was safe from one of Mark's hilarious practical jokes. Over the years, his friends Tom, Jen, and Sarah had endured it all - from whoopee cushions to scary clown masks to finding their cars on blocks.

But this year, they decided it was time for some sweet revenge on Mark's upcoming 30th birthday. As they brainstormed ideas over beer and pizza one night, the plan started coming together.

"We need to up the ante, go all out if we want to one-up Mark," said Tom.

"How about we hide his car in a massive storage unit across town?" suggested Jen.

Sarah shook her head. "Nah, too mean. We need funny, not malicious."

A devious smile spread across Tom's face. "I've got it... We'll tell him we're having a birthday dinner as usual. But when he shows up..."

On the big day, Mark was suspicious when all his friends blew him off with vague excuses about being "busy". But when 7 pm rolled around and he still hadn't heard anything, he started to get a little worried and hurt. Did they forget his birthday?

Just then, his phone rang. "Hey man, so sorry for the confusion. Dinner is actually at my place tonight. See you in 20?" said Tom.

When Mark arrived at Tom's, he found the house completely dark and silent. "Hello? Guys? Very funny joke..." he called out as he stepped inside.

Suddenly, the lights flipped on to reveal his friends crammed into the tiny foyer, wearing rubber gorilla masks and making loud monkey noises. Mark screamed and nearly jumped out of his skin.

"HA! Gotcha!" they all hollered in unison while ripping off their masks, cackling with laughter at the success of their prank.

"Not bad, very spooky," admitted Mark with a grin, "Now where's the real party?"

Tom smirked. "The party's just getting started, my friend." He led Mark into the kitchen, which was empty except for a single plate on the center island. On it sat a small cupcake with a sparkler candle flickering.

"HAPPY BIRTHDAY!!" his friends shouted as Mark's jaw dropped in shock and amusement.

"No way...you guys emptied the kitchen for one sad cupcake?" he laughed.

"Check the pantry," said Jen mischievously.

Mark pulled open the pantry door to find it stuffed to the brim with snacks, drinks, and a gorgeous three-tier cake overflowing with frosting roses.

"We got you, you pranking jerk!" cackled Sarah.

The rest of the night was filled with laughter, inside jokes, memories, and of course, plenty of cake. As it turned out, revenge was sweet - but not as sweet as the joy of celebrating with friends, and having a few good laughs along the way. Mark decided then and there that he'd finally met his match, and was proud to pass the pranking torch. Because getting played at your own game? Now that's the best kind of payback.

Title: "A Perfect Harmony"

Sara sighed as she packed up her guitar after another long rehearsal with her band. They had a big show coming up at the local bar and still hadn't nailed down their setlist. As much as she loved singing and performing, being in a band could be stressful at times.

"Great work tonight everyone," said their lead guitarist and bandleader, Dylan. "I think we're starting to come together. A few more practices and we'll be ready to rock the Block Party!" The rest of the band cheered in agreement, though Sara couldn't help but stare at Dylan as he packed up his guitar.

Ever since joining the band six months ago, Sara had developed a bit of a crush on Dylan. With his shaggy brown hair, leather jacket, and effortless guitar skills, it was easy to see why all the girls swooned over him. The problem was that Dylan had a long-term girlfriend, Jenna, who was practically attached to his hip at all times. Sara knew her feelings were silly and pointless, but she couldn't help it – there was just something about Dylan's passion for music that drew her to him.

In the weeks leading up to the show, Sara found herself getting closer and closer to Dylan as they worked on song arrangements and rehearsed together after band practice. Dylan was a natural leader and teacher – he had a gift for bringing out the best in all the musicians. Sara loved learning from him and getting his feedback on her vocals. Late one night after a marathon three-hour rehearsal, the two found themselves alone at the studio sharing a pizza.

"You're coming into your own as a frontwoman, Sara," Dylan said through a mouthful of cheese. "Your voice has so much emotion and power behind it. The band is lucky to have you."

Sara blushed at the compliment. "Thanks, that means a lot coming from you. I'm just trying to keep up with the rest of you talented guys."

They continued chatting about music and their hopes for the band's future. Before Sara knew it, it was past midnight. "I should probably get going," she said with a yawn. "Got work in the morning."

"Let me walk you out," said Dylan, ever the gentleman. As they reached Sara's car, he lingered by her door. "Thanks again for all your hard work, Sara. The band really wouldn't be the same without you."

At that moment, staring into Dylan's kind eyes under the glow of the streetlamp, Sara felt her heart pounding. Without thinking, she leaned in and kissed him softly on the lips. Dylan froze, clearly taken by surprise. But instead of pulling away, he kissed her back...

To be continued! I hope you enjoyed the start of this story touching on the prompt you provided. Let me know if you'd like me to continue the tale of Sara, Dylan, and the band's journey towards love, music, and that all-important show!

Title: "A Tooth Hurts but Love Heals"

Jenna had a terrible fear of dentists ever since a bad experience as a child. So when a painful toothache started keeping her up at night, she put off making an appointment as long as she could. Finally, the pain was just too much and she reluctantly called her local dental office.

Luckily, they had a cancellation and could get her in that afternoon. As she sat nervously in the waiting room, she started having second thoughts about coming. But then she heard a kind voice call her name. "Jenna Roberts?"

When she looked up, she was surprised by how good-looking her dentist was. Dr. Adam Smith had a warm smile that immediately put her at ease. "Thanks for squeezing me in on such short notice," Jenna said as she followed him back.

"Not a problem at all. Now, let's take a look at that painful tooth." Much to Jenna's surprise, she didn't find the dentist visit too bad. Adam was very gentle and reassuring. Within no time, he had found the problem - a bad cavity. "I'm afraid it will need a root canal. But don't worry, we'll get you all fixed up."

Over the next few weeks, Jenna returned to Adam's office for the root canal and crown procedure. Along the way, she found herself looking forward to her visits...not because of the dental work, but because she enjoyed chatting with Adam. His kind manner had helped ease her fear.

Before she knew it, her dental issues were resolved. But Jenna realized she wasn't ready to stop seeing the dentist she had grown so fond of. Mustering up her courage, she asked Adam out for coffee. To her delight, he accepted with a smile. Their coffee date turned into dinner and then many more dates after that.

Jenna was amazed at how someone she initially dreaded, a dentist, had become the man who helped her overcome her fears and stolen her heart. Adam was happy he could not only help fix Jenna's tooth but also mend her broken heart. Their chance meeting in the dental chair led to a love that would continue making them smile for years to come.

Title: "Nanny Nanette Nabs the Senator"

Jill Jackson was fed up with her dead-end job answering phones at a small tabloid newspaper. She wanted to do some real investigative journalism and expose corruption. When rumors started circulating about a high-profile senator who was mistreating his staff, Jill saw her chance.

She applied for a job posting as a live-in nanny for the senator's three kids. During the interview, the frazzled wife complained about how busy the senator was and how hard it was to find good help. Jill played up her childcare skills and experience. On the surface, she seemed like the perfect candidate.

Jill got the job and moved into the spacious but chaotic house. The three kids, ages 5 to 10, had no boundaries or discipline. Jill worked hard to establish routines and structure during the day. At night, she dug through papers and listened at doors when she could, hoping to find evidence of the senator's alleged misdeeds.

After a few weeks, Jill had nothing solid. The kids were improving under her care but the senator always seemed to avoid being home. Then one night, Jill overheard a loud argument between the senator and his wife. She heard him accuse his wife of snooping around his desk. When Jill heard a crash, she burst into the room to find the wife crying on the floor beside an overturned table.

Jill helped the wife upstairs and then called the local women's shelter for advice. They told her to quietly document any instances of abuse to build a case. A few nights later, Jill witnessed the senator push his wife against the kitchen counter during another fight. She secretly snapped photos on her phone, the first hard proof she had found.

The next day, Jill sat down with the kids and had a thoughtful discussion about treating all people, including parents, with kindness and respect. That evening, the oldest boy told Jill he didn't feel safe with his dad sometimes. Jill's heart broke for the family. She knew she needed to act fast to protect them.

That weekend, Jill waited for the senator to leave on one of his "business trips." She searched his office more thoroughly this time and discovered receipts documenting thousands of dollars in personal expenses billed to his campaign fund. Eureka! Jill made copies of everything before returning the papers neatly.

She anonymously sent her evidence to the newspaper and women's groups. Within days, allegations of embezzlement and domestic violence were swirling around the senator. With mounting public pressure and actual victims coming forward, he had no choice but to resign from office.

Jill left her job as a nanny, no longer needing the cover. She handed over all her research and photos to the newspaper, finally getting her big break. Her exposé won awards, and she was offered a reporting job at a major city paper. Sometime later, she reunited with the now-divorced family. The children had thrived under Jill's care, and the wife was getting counseling. They thanked Jill for her courage in standing up to the corrupt politician when no one else would. Her story helped others find the strength to speak out as well. Another victory for truth and justice, thanks to Nanny Nanette!

Title: "How Bob The Puppy Saved Me From Myself"

Samantha had always been more of a cat person. She saw dogs as dirty, slobbery creatures that were too dependent on their owners. Give her a quiet, independent cat any day.

When her neighbor Mary suddenly had to move abroad for a new job, she was desperate to find a home for her eight-month-old Labrador, Bob. Despite Samantha's protests, Mary begged her to look after him for a few weeks until she could make other arrangements. What else could Samantha say but yes?

The first night with Bob was a disaster. He cried and howled in his crate no matter what Samantha did. He chewed up her favorite shoes and knocked over every lamp chasing his tail. By morning, Samantha was exhausted and convinced this was a mistake.

Over the next few days though, Bob began to win her over with his enthusiasm and good nature. He seemed to know just when to cheer her up with a lick on the hand or cuddle on the couch. Soon that slobbery tongue was bringing a smile instead of a scowl.

Samantha started to look forward to their walks in the park each evening. Bob would bound over to every person and dog, wanting to make as many new friends as possible. His joy was infectious. Strangers would smile and wave at Samantha now too, even striking up conversations about her adorable pup. She found herself chatting with the other dog owners, surprised at how friendly a community it was. For the first time in ages, she didn't feel so alone.

One weekend, Samantha's friend Jessica was visiting. While they sat in the garden enjoying the sunshine, Bob bounded up with his favorite rope toy, begging for a game. "I don't know how you do it, keeping up with that bundle of energy!" laughed Jessica. But Samantha realized with surprise that playing with Bob didn't feel like a chore - it had become one of the highlights of her day.

A few more weeks went by and still no word from Mary about taking Bob back. Samantha knew she should be contacting other potential homes, but the thought of giving him up was unbearable. This lovable pup had made his way into her heart like no other.

One morning as they walked, Bob stopped suddenly and whimpered, pawing at something on the ground. Samantha peered over and gasped - it was an elderly man who had collapsed. She called 999 immediately and stayed with the man until the ambulance arrived. As he was loaded onto the stretcher, he grasped Samantha's hand. "Thank you...my dog never would have found me in time. You and your pup saved my life today."

That's when it hit Samantha - Bob had a gift for knowing when someone needed help. And in the process of rescuing that man, he had rescued her too from her loneliness. This dog had changed her life in more ways than she ever thought possible. He was family now, and she couldn't imagine her world without him in it.

A few days later, Mary called to say she was permanently relocating overseas and offered to sign Bob over to Samantha. Her answer was a joyful "Yes!" And so it was that a woman who once hated dogs ended up with the best dog of all, who taught her that love and companionship can come in unexpected places when you open your heart. Bob would be by her side from that day on, helping her see the world - and herself - in a whole new light.

Title: "A Sneezy Surprise"

John was not having the best day. He woke up with a stuffy nose and itchy, watery eyes. "Not again," he thought to himself. John was severely allergic to most flowers, especially roses, but someone had decided to play a prank on him. When he walked outside to get the mail, there sitting on his front porch was a gorgeous bouquet of two dozen red roses.

He sneezed just looking at them. Through watery eyes, he spotted an envelope tucked amongst the blooms. "Who on earth would send me flowers?" he wondered as another massive sneeze overtook him. Wiping his nose on his sleeve, he plucked the envelope free. Inside was a short note written in elegant script:

"Dear John,

I've admired you from afar for too long. Please join me for coffee this Saturday at 2 pm so I can finally introduce myself. I hope you enjoy the flowers, even if they do make you sneezy.

Your Secret Admirer"

John's heart jumped in his chest. A secret admirer? Someone was interested in him? But who? And how did they not know about his terrible allergies? Another sneeze wracked his body as the pollen from the roses filled the air. He had to get these flowers inside, away from his sensitive nose and eyes.

Gingerly picking up the bouquet, he carried them through the front door while trying not to breathe through his nose. Once safely inside, he fetched an empty vase, filled it with water, and arranged the roses. Even from across the room, he could feel another sneezing fit coming on. His eyes were so watery and puffy he could barely see.

"I hope this coffee date is worth it," he grumbled as he fetched a handful of tissues. The next two days dragged on as John's allergies raged. Nothing seemed to soothe his poor nose and eyes. By Saturday morning, he looked an absolute mess. His normally clear complexion was now red and blotchy from endless sneezing. But he didn't want to disappoint his secret admirer by standing them up.

Just after 2 pm, John shuffled into the busy coffee shop, tissues stuffed up both sleeves just in case. He scanned the tables, hoping to spot someone waving at him. Instead, he was greeted by a chipper voice behind the counter. "John? I'm so glad you could make it!" The barista beamed at him with a bright smile.

"Sarah?" John cringed, realizing his stuffy voice probably sounded terrible. Sarah had been his barista for over a year. Every morning he came in for his regular coffee and they would chat. She was bubbly and funny, always brightening his day. But he had no idea she felt anything more than friendly coworker vibes.

Sarah blushed and slipped out from behind the counter. "I know, I know. The flowers probably weren't the best idea for your allergies. But I had to do something to get your attention!" John suddenly didn't feel quite so stuffy. His heart swelled knowing someone as wonderful as Sarah returned his feelings.

"You got my attention alright," he chuckled, then sneezed loudly into a tissue. "And I think my allergies will survive one coffee date with you." Sarah beamed and took his hand. As they sat down to chat, brewing cups of coffee forgotten, John decided maybe flowers weren't so bad after all...if they led him to love.

Title: "Facing Her Fears for Love"

Sara couldn't believe she agreed to do this. As she watched the hot air balloon being prepared for takeoff, her heart felt like it was in her throat. She had a deathly fear of heights ever since she was a little girl. But when her long-time crush Jack had asked her on a romantic hot air balloon ride for their first official date, she didn't have the heart to say no.

Sara had liked Jack from afar for over a year now but never dared to tell him how she felt. When he finally asked her out last week, she was over the moon. But now, as she watched the basket being loaded with champagne, flower petals, and a picnic basket for their evening ride, she started to seriously regret her decision.

"Nervous?" Jack asked sweetly, coming up behind her and placing a reassuring hand on her shoulder. Sara jumped slightly at his touch.

"Is it that obvious?" She asked with a shaky laugh.

"It's okay, I'll be right there to hold your hand the whole time. You'll be safe with me, I promise." Jack said with a warm smile.

Sara smiled back, already feeling herself calming down a bit in his presence. There was just something about Jack that made her feel at ease. Maybe facing her fear of the chance of love would be worth it.

"Alright, everyone, we're all set for takeoff!" called the pilot. "You two lovebirds hop on in."

Jack held out his hand for Sara. She took a deep breath and placed her shaky hand in his steady one. He gave it a gentle, reassuring squeeze as he helped her climb into the basket. Sara did her best not to look over the edge as she sat down. Jack sat right next to her and kept a hold of her hand.

"Ready for an evening you'll never forget?" He asked with a charming grin. Sara smiled and nodded, trying to ignore the nerves bouncing around in her stomach.

The pilot lit the propane burner under the balloon and they slowly started to rise into the air. Sara gasped and gripped Jack's hand tighter as she felt the ground move farther away beneath her. Jack just smiled and rubbed comforting circles on the back of her hand with his thumb.

"Look, isn't it beautiful?" He asked in awe, gesturing to the breathtaking view with his free hand.

Sara cautiously peeked over the edge of the basket and her breath caught in her throat. They were high enough now to see for miles in every direction as the sun was starting to set over the horizon, painting the sky in gorgeous pinks, oranges, and purples. Fields, forests, and the twinkling city lights down below looked like a postcard come to life. Even the pilot was silenced by the sheer natural magnificence surrounding them.

"It's...it's amazing," Sara said softly. And in that moment, she realized she wasn't scared anymore. With Jack by her side and the picture before her, any fear she once had completely melted away.

They spent the next hour floating gently through the sky, feeding each other chocolate-covered strawberries and sipping champagne as the stars began to shine brighter than Sara had ever seen before. Jack pointed out different constellations and shared cute astronomy facts with her. Before she knew it, two bottles of champagne and the entire picnic basket were gone.

"Thank you for bringing me up here tonight, Jack. I'll never forget this as long as I live." Sara said sincerely as the pilot started their descent back to land.

"You're very welcome, Sara. I'm so glad you decided to face your fear. I think you're incredibly brave." Jack said, giving her a loving look that made her heart skip a beat.

When they touched down safely back on the ground, Sara was surprised to realize she wasn't afraid or uneasy at all. She was sad the magical night was over. Jack walked her to her front door, and they paused outside, still holding hands.

"I like you, Sara. Will you go out with me again?" Jack asked hopefully.

Sara smiled brilliantly, feeling like the luckiest girl in the world. "Absolutely. I think I'm starting to like you too."

They shared their first sweet kiss under the moonlight as fireworks seemed to erupt inside Sara's heart. Maybe facing fears was worth it after all, if it led her to falling deeply in love.

Title: "Checkmate, Grandpa"

Young Billy couldn't wait to get home from school. At only 10 years old, he had shown such natural talent and skill at chess that his teacher had entered him into several local tournaments, where he had emerged victorious against kids much older than him. Billy's grandfather, Pop, had taught him how to play when he was just 5. Ever since they spent every Friday night together huddled over the chessboard in the den.

But tonight was different. Tonight, Billy was going to challenge Pop to a game. All the other kids he had beaten were amateurs compared to Pop, whom Billy had never actually played against. Pop had gone undefeated in his town's senior center chess club tournaments for over a decade. Billy was confident in his abilities now though. He just knew he had improved enough to take down the old man.

When Billy burst through the front door, dropping his backpack by the stairs, Pop was already setting up the board in the den like always. But tonight, the piece placement felt different, more serious somehow.

"You ready for our first official match, champ?" Pop asked, not looking up from centering the king and queen.

Billy felt butterflies erupt in his stomach but steeled his nerves. "You bet I am, Pop. I've been practicing nonstop. I think I'm finally ready to beat you."

Pop just chuckled, his belly shaking. "We'll see about that, Billy boy. I've been playing this game a long time before you were even born!"

The game began tentatively as they both felt each other out, neither wanting to make the first mistake. But soon, Billy started gaining momentum, taking Pop's pieces with calculated precision. He had always been such a methodical player. Within 30 minutes, it was obvious Billy had Pop on the ropes. Only a few pieces remained on the board for each of them.

Watching his grandson play, Pop felt a swell of pride in his chest. His old heart could barely contain it. He had never seen anyone, especially not a kid Billy's age, play with such natural skill and smarts. It was then that Pop realized the time had come for a life lesson that was much bigger than just a chess game.

On Billy's next turn, Pop deliberately left himself open and bowed his head, "Checkmate, my boy. You got me fair and square."

"What? No way!" Billy cried, surveying the board in disbelief. But sure enough, his king was cornered with no escape. He had won.

Pop met Billy's bewildered eyes with a sad smile. "I concede defeat, Billy. You are truly a great player."

Confused, Billy asked, "But Pop, why'd you let me win? I thought this was a real match!"

Pop sighed heavily as he began putting the pieces gently back into their velvet bags. "Oh, it was very real, son. Make no mistake - you beat me honestly with your talent and skill. But I wanted to teach you something more important than just the game."

He paused, gathering his thoughts. "You see, Billy, in life, it's not always about who wins or loses. What matters is how we treat each other, especially family, along the way. I'm so proud of the player you've become, and I wanted you to know that."

Overcome, Billy threw his arms around Pop's broad shoulders. He had never quite understood the depth of Pop's wisdom until that moment. A game was just a game, but family was forever.

"Thanks for teaching me Pop, both chess and life's big lessons. You'll always be the champion in my book."

Pop ruffled Billy's hair, eyes glistening. "And you'll always be my champ too, son. Now, how about some ice cream to celebrate? I think we've both earned it!"

Title: "Catfished Hearts"

Jake was nervous as he got into his car, ready to drive two hours to meet Hannah for the first time in person. They had been chatting online for the past six months and connected. Hannah seemed perfect - she was beautiful, funny, and so easy to talk to. Jake thought this could be something special.

As Jake drove, he started to feel uneasy. Hannah's photos were from a few years ago and on her profile, it said she was in great shape. What if she had let herself go lately? Jake didn't have recent photos posted either, as he was also a few years old. He had gained some weight since then but hoped Hannah wouldn't notice or care too much. All Jake could do was hope for the best and continue to meet her.

When Jake arrived at the cafe they agreed to meet at, he took a deep breath before walking in. He scanned the room and didn't see Hannah at first, but then caught sight of a larger woman waving at him from a corner booth. It was her. Jake put on a smile and walked over, hoping she wouldn't notice his hesitation.

"Hi Hannah, it's so nice to finally meet you!" Jake said as he hugged her. Her photos didn't do justice to how much weight she had gained. She filled out the booth, and her double chin was prominent as she smiled widely at him.

"Jake! I'm so happy to see you in person," Hannah giggled. "Wow, you clean up nicely! Your photos must be a few years old too, huh?" she commented, staring at his fuller frame.

They chatted awkwardly at first as they both noticed the differences from the pictures. As they talked more, though, Jake found himself laughing and enjoying Hannah's company just as much as online. Her witty sense of humor and kind spirit shone through, just as before. Pretty soon, Jake forgot all about her appearance and was fully engaged in their conversation.

A couple of hours passed by without them even noticing. The café was starting to empty as closing time neared.

"I can't believe how late it's gotten! This has been so fun; I'm glad we finally did this," Hannah said with a sigh.

"Me too. I know our photos didn't exactly match up to current reality, but I'm really glad I came," Jake smiled. "I feel like we have an even stronger connection in person. Would you like to get dinner sometime?"

A look of relief and joy washed over Hannah's face. "I'd love that. And maybe next time we can exchange more recent pictures so there are no surprises," she laughed.

Jake laughed with her, feeling content. Looks had been deceiving when it came to Hannah, but her heart was as beautiful on the inside as he hoped. What started with white lies online had blossomed into something real and caring right in front of them. Jake was thankful that despite the catfishing, they found an honesty and bond deeper than any photograph could show. It seemed they both had found what they were searching for.

Title: "Love Behind the Face Paint"

Sally had been a professional clown for over 20 years. She loved making people laugh and spreading joy, even if it meant wearing hilarious colorful costumes and oversized shoes. What she didn't love was how terrifying clowns seemed to be for some people. She had heard of this phobia known as coulrophobia but never thought she'd meet someone who had it.

That all changed one day when Sally was booked to perform at the city park's summer carnival. As she was getting ready in her trailer, applying her signature bright red nose and face paint, she overheard two couples talking nearby. One man seemed on edge as his friend was trying to convince him to check out the clown show. "Come on John, the kids will love it! It's just a clown." John replied nervously, "You know I can't stand those things; they give me the creeps."

Sally decided to introduce herself, hoping to ease John's mind about clowns before the show. As she approached, John looked like a scared rabbit ready to bolt at any moment when he saw her face paint and colorful wig. "Hi there! No need to be afraid, I come in peace. My name is Sally and I promise the show is only filled with laughter, no creeps involved." John was still clearly uncomfortable but smiled politely. "I'm John. Nice to meet you...I think."

The longer they talked, the more Sally found herself enchanted by John's kind eyes and handsome smile beneath his nerves. By the end of her show, which featured pratfalls, balloon animals, and sight gags, John was even laughing alongside the kids despite still keeping his distance from Sally in her full clown getup. A spark had been ignited between them.

Over the following weeks, Sally and John continued to run into each other at the park as Sally's clowning duties brought her around regularly. Her feelings grew stronger with each chance encounter, but she struggled with how to pursue anything knowing of his unease with clowns. That was until one sunny afternoon, John spotted Sally out of her clown outfit for a rare time, just wearing jeans and a t-shirt as she took a break to eat lunch. "Sally? Is that you under there?" he asked with a smile.

They shared their first real conversation without any face paint or costumes getting in the way. Sally told John more about how much she loved making people happy through clowning and John opened up about how a scary clown attacked him as a child, sparking the phobia he still lived with. But being with Sally, he realized not all clowns were bad and perhaps his fear was something he wanted to overcome if it meant having a chance with her.

Each day after that, John joined Sally for her breaks as they got to know each other better beyond colorful wigs and oversized shoes. Slowly but surely, his fear faded more and more into the background. Finally, one sunny afternoon a few months later, John took a deep breath, walked right up to Sally in full clown attire, and placed a gentle kiss on her cheek behind the face paint. "I think I'm ready to give this clown-loving girl of my dreams a try if she'll have me."

Sally grinned from ear to ear, both natural and painted-on, as she embraced him. "She most definitely will." And so a true love began between an unlikely pair who proved that happiness can be found even in the most surprising of places and that fears are best faced together hand in hand with someone who cares. They lived, as the saying goes, happily ever after.

Title: "A Tasty Surprise for Herbivore Heart"

Jake was nervous as he pulled up to Sarah's house to pick her up for their first date. She was gorgeous and he wanted to impress her. But there was one problem - Sarah was a die-hard carnivore who loved a juicy steak, while Jake had been a vegan chef for the past 5 years.

When they got to the restaurant, Sarah smiled as she looked over the menu. "I think I'll get the 16oz ribeye with mashed potatoes. It looks amazing!" Jake gulped, wishing he had chosen a vegan spot for their date. But he wanted Sarah to experience his cooking, so he had decided to cook her dinner himself back at his place.

As they drove back to Jake's apartment, he kept thinking of excuses for what he was about to serve. "I hope you like pasta...with tomatoes...and carrots...no meat whatsoever!" But Sarah just laughed. "Don't worry Jake, I keep an open mind about food. I'm sure it will be delicious no matter what."

They arrived at his apartment which was filled with the aroma of something simmering. Jake led Sarah to the kitchen, nervous for her reaction. But to his surprise, on the stove was a sizzling steak, cooked to perfection, alongside roasted potatoes and sautéed mushrooms. "Jake! How...I thought you were vegan?" Sarah gasped.

Jake chuckled. "I am, but I wanted to cook something I knew you'd love. Turns out, with the right spices and a little olive oil, even a vegan can grill up an impressive steak. I hope you like it!" Sarah took a bite and her eyes rolled back with pleasure. "This is better than any steak I've ever had before! You'll have to give me the recipe. And any man who can cook like this...well, I think we'll be having a second date!"

So even though he was a vegan chef, Jake proved to his carnivore date that meat didn't have to come from an animal to be truly tasty. It was a surprising success, and just might have been the start of something special between them!

Title: "The Theorem of Beauty"

Jane was always told she was smart but never beautiful. As the top of her class in math and science, she excelled at theorems but not at popularity contests. So when the local beauty pageant came to town, hosted by the town's biggest cheerleading squad no less, she got an idea.

"I'll enter that pageant and show them that beauty is more than just looks," she told her friend Algebra (yes really, that was his name). Algebra thought she was crazy but knew better than to argue.

On the big night, Jane dazzled the crowd with her math theorems and formulas, proving various geometric principles with equations written all over her sash. The other girls looked on confused, trying to remember their 5-word talent answers to simple questions.

When it came time for the question portion, Jane was ready. "So tell me Miss Math, how would you improve our education system?" asked the host cheerleader. Without missing a beat, Jane launched into a passionate explanation involving pie charts and standard deviations showing statistical proof that increased STEM funding leads to higher test scores and more college degrees. The host had no choice but to nod along, even if she didn't understand a word of it.

Somehow, Jane's unique approach started to win people over. Her enthusiasm and intelligence shone through in a way raw beauty could not. Even the host had to admit, there was more to this girl than met the eye.

When the final results were read, Jane was shocked to hear her name called the new beauty queen. But she knew that true beauty was what was inside, and she had proven her point. Sometimes the most unexpected people can change our views if we only open our minds beyond the surface. And sometimes, the perfect formula for success has variables we'd never think to include.

Title: "The Accidental Spy Next Door"

James had always worked as a spy for years, going undercover on dangerous missions all over the world. But he was getting burnt out from all the secrecy and deception. He longed for a normal life where he didn't have to hide who he truly was.

That all changed when the beautiful Melissa moved in next door. James was instantly smitten with her kind smile and bubbly laughter. He wanted nothing more than to ask her out, but how could he reveal his real job to her? She'd never understand the dangers of his world.

So James decided to try living a normal life for once. He quit his spy job and got work at the local hardware store. Every morning he'd smile and wave to Melissa, striking up cheerful conversations about the neighborhood or the latest movies. Melissa seemed to enjoy his company.

One weekend, Melissa was working on a home renovation project and was struggling to put together a new cabinet set she had purchased. James happened to be outside gardening and overheard her frustrated curses through the open window.

He volunteered to come help, bringing along his toolbox. "It's just a side hobby of mine to work on home projects," James said casually as he efficiently assembled the cabinet in no time. Melissa was impressed by his skills.

As they talked, Melissa let slip that she had tickets to the county fair that weekend but her date had bailed. James saw his chance and asked if she'd like to go with him instead. Melissa smiled and said yes.

The county fair was in full swing when they arrived. James won Melissa a giant teddy bear at the basketball toss. As they walked around, James told amusing anecdotes about fictional mishaps from past home renovations. Melissa was enthralled by his stories and easy humor.

They shared a fun afternoon until suddenly James recognized two men lurking in the crowd as known assassins from his past missions. He realized with dread that his cover may have been compromised. Worse, Melissa was now in danger too since she was with him.

"I apologize Melissa, but I have to tell you the truth. Those men over there, they're very dangerous. I used to work covert operations taking down guys like them. But I wanted a normal life, which is why I'm here with you now."

Melissa stared at him, understandably shocked. But to James' surprise, she smiled. "You know, I had a hunch there was more to you than meets the eye. I appreciate you being honest with me now. And for what it's worth...I think you make a great spy AND a great neighbor."

James breathed a sigh of relief. Maybe his two worlds didn't have to be so separate after all. And with Melissa by his side, he felt ready to take on any danger that came his way. It just went to show, you never know what life has in store when you least expect it.

Title: "A Second Chance at Love"

Sophie couldn't believe it when she saw the name on the wedding planning inquiry. It had been 5 years since she last heard from her ex Jacob, and now he was getting married and wanted to hire her company to plan the event.

Their breakup had been painful - they seemed so in love and had even talked about getting married someday themselves. But then Jacob got a big promotion at work that required him to move across the country. Neither of them wanted to do long distance, so they sadly decided to end things. Sophie was heartbroken for months.

Now here was Jacob's name in her inbox. She almost didn't want to take the job, worried it would just open old wounds. But her curiosity got the best of her and she decided to at least meet with him to discuss the job.

When Jacob walked into her office, Sophie's heart skipped a beat just like it used to. He looked just as handsome as she remembered. They made some small talk, catching up on the last 5 years of their lives. Jacob explained that his fiance Allison loved Sophie's work and wanted her specifically to plan the wedding.

As they discussed wedding details, Sophie was surprised by how comfortable and natural it felt to be with Jacob again. Old feelings started bubbling up that she thought were long buried. But she had to professionally focus on the task at hand.

Over the next few months of planning, Sophie and Jacob grew even closer. They fell back into an easy rhythm with each other as they tasted cakes, tried food samples, and visited possible venues together. Allison was busy with work and often couldn't attend planning meetings. Jacob and Sophie would look at wedding magazines for hours, laughing and remembering their dreams from years ago.

It became harder and harder for Sophie to separate her work relationship from the romantic past she still cared for deeply. One night after a few glasses of wine during a planning meeting, their feelings boiled over. They kissed passionately, realizing the fire between them never truly went away. But it was followed by regret and guilt.

Jacob admitted he still had feelings for Sophie too, but he was committed to Allison. Sophie realized she couldn't continue working on the wedding anymore. It was simply too hard and confusing to her heart. They said their goodbyes, leaving things unfinished once again.

On the day of the big wedding, Sophie couldn't help but feel heartbroken seeing Jacob marry another woman. She wondered if they would ever find their way back to each other. But then just before the ceremony, Jacob came running down the aisle. "I'm sorry, I can't do this. I'm still in love with you Sophie," he declared.

The guests gasped as Jacob brought Sophie up to the altar instead. In that moment, they both knew their love was as strong as ever and they were meant to be together after all. Sophie would get her happy ending as a bride instead of just the wedding planner this time around.

Title: "The Case of Kris Kringle vs The Prosecution"

Jennifer Smythe sighed as she reviewed the case file on her desk. As one of the top defense lawyers in the city, she handled all sorts of criminal cases from drug runners to murderers. But this case was like nothing she had ever seen before. Her new client, a 64-year-old man named Kris Kringle, was insisting that he was, in fact, Santa Claus and was being charged with public disturbance, resisting arrest, and fraud.

When Jennifer had first taken the call from Kris, she thought it was some prank. But after meeting with him, she could sense he genuinely believed he was Santa. Perhaps he had some delusions or was playing a very committed prank, but he did not seem dangerous or malicious. Jennifer decided to take the case, more as a curiosity than anything else.

On the day of the trial, Jennifer strode into the courtroom, briefcase in hand. She took a seat next to Kris and gave him a reassuring nod. "Just stay calm and let me do the talking, OK Kris?" He nodded solemnly in return.

The prosecution began by outlining how Kris had been found standing on a street corner in full Santa costume on a hot summer's day, insisting to passersby that he was "checking his list" and taking down names of those who were naughty and nice. When police approached him to move him along, he started yelling about how "Rudolph would trample them if they didn't watch it" and had to be forcibly restrained.

During the prosecution's testimony, Kris shook his head vigorously. "Objection your honor, these lies will not do. I am attempting to do my important work, even in the summer solstice when the Christmas spirit is needed most." The judge glared at Kris. "Mr Kringle, let your lawyer do the talking please."

When it was Jennifer's turn, she addressed the court calmly. "Ladies and gentlemen, while my client Kris may have some unconventional beliefs, he is a gentle soul who means no harm. Perhaps in his mind, he was simply spreading some Christmas cheer during a hot summer, unaware of how unusual his actions seemed. But he did not threaten or assault anyone. At worst this was a misunderstanding between a fanciful man and the laws of public disturbance. I ask that you show compassion and drop all charges."

During the recess, Jennifer visited Kris. "Just hang in there a little longer. I think I may have swayed the jury in our favor." Kris smiled his kind old smile. "Bless you, Jennifer, for believing in an old man like me. And bless all people for finding the Christmas spirit within, whatever the time of year." His warmth and sincerity moved even the tough lawyer.

When the court reconvened, the jury took only a short time to come back with their verdict. "Not guilty on all charges." The judge banged his gavel. "Case dismissed." As Kris and Jennifer left the courtroom together, reporters swarmed, wanting to hear from the "real" Santa Claus.

"No more words from me today," said Kris gently. "Just remember that Christmas lives in every one of our hearts, every day of the year, if we care for each other and spread love as I strive to do." Jennifer watched Kris go with a new respect for the elderly man. Maybe he wasn't Santa biologically, but in spirit he surely was. And sometimes that's what matters.

Title: "Rock Star Undercover"

Johnny Steel was exhausted from being on tour for the past year as the lead singer of the chart-topping rock band "Metal Mayhem". While he loved performing for crowds of adoring fans, the hectic schedule and constant limelight had started to wear him down. He desperately needed a break from it all.

One night after a big show, Johnny had too much to drink and started joking with his bandmates about how entertaining it would be to go undercover at a high school and experience what "normal" teenagers dealt with every day. To his surprise, the rest of the guys thought it was a great idea and encouraged Johnny to go through with it.

After sobering up, Johnny began to seriously consider the plan. He dyed his long hair brown, grew some stubble on his face, and packed up some suits and ties to complete his disguise. With the help of some forged documents, Johnny was able to get a substitute teaching position at the local public high school.

On Johnny's first day, he was nervous but excited to start his undercover adventure. He introduced himself as "Mr. Smith" to his freshman English class. Throughout the day, Johnny was surprised by how rowdy and disrespectful some of the students were towards their teachers. He also couldn't believe how distracted the kids were by their phones!

Johnny began to gain the students' respect as he demonstrated his extensive knowledge of literature and gave engaging lessons. He also surprised the football team by joining in for practice and showing off his incredible strength and agility from years of performing. Word started spreading around the school about their coolest sub, "Mr. Smith".

During his time undercover, Johnny realized he loved helping the students discover new interests and guiding them toward their potential. He also found joy in the simple things he had been missing like laughing with friends at a high school basketball game. By the end of the term, Johnny had become quite fond of his teaching job and the community within the school.

As Johnny was preparing for his last day, the principal came to him with a proposal. "Mr. Smith, the English department head position is opening up next year and we'd love for you to apply. Will you consider becoming a full-time teacher here?" Johnny smiled, knowing he had found his new calling in life, away from the madness of the rock star world. He graciously accepted the position, ready to trade in his microphone for a teacher's magic marker.

Title: "Tooth Hurts and the Heart"

Dr. Sarah Wilson has been a dentist for 10 years now. She loved her work and took great joy in helping people overcome their dental fears. One day a new patient named John Smith came in, trembling with nerves. "Relax, I don't bite!" Sarah joked, trying to lighten the mood. But John seemed beyond terrified.

Throughout a few appointments, Sarah gently worked on gaining John's trust while also fixing his dental issues. "You're doing so well," she kept encouraging. Through it all, Sarah found herself thinking more and more about John's warm smile and kind eyes. Was she developing feelings for a patient? She tried to ignore her racing heartbeat whenever John entered the room.

Once his treatment was over, John thanked Sarah profusely. "It's my job to help people with their dental health. I'm just glad you're not afraid anymore," she said with a smile. But to her surprise, John spoke up. "I may not be afraid of the dentist anymore, but now I'm afraid of something else. I think I'm falling for my dentist."

Sarah's heart skipped a beat. Was this happening? They decided to start slow, with casual dates outside of the dental office. Over coffee, long walks in the park, and funny conversations, they realized their connection went far deeper than patient and doctor. Sarah had helped John overcome his fear, and in the process, he had helped her overcome her fears about mixing work with romance.

A year later, John came in for his regular dental cleaning. But this time, he got down on one knee instead. With tears in her eyes, Sarah said "yes" right there in the exam room. Their hearts had found each other through courage, compassion, and a little bit of tooth therapy. It just went to show - love can happen when you least expect it, even between a dentist and her patient.

Title: "Family Vacation from Hell"

Jane sighed as she packed her suitcase. A forced vacation was the last thing she wanted to do right now; she had so many projects at work to finish up. But her boss was insistent, telling her she was working too many hours and needed to unplug.

So here she was, packing for a week at her parents' beach house with her parents, two sisters, and all of their families in tow. Jane's relationship with her family had become increasingly distant over the years as her career took off. While they all still got along on the surface, they didn't know each other anymore.

Jane drove the three hours to the beach house feeling anxious the whole way. She wasn't sure how she was going to survive a whole week living in close quarters with her family without tearing her hair out. As she pulled into the driveway, she steeled herself for what was to come.

Her mother greeted her warmly at the door, seeming genuinely happy to see her. "We're so glad you could make it, Jane! It's been too long since we've all been together." Jane returned the greeting as enthusiastically as she could muster.

Her sisters were there with their husbands and kids. Jane watched them all interacting together happily and felt a pang of sadness and jealousy at the relationships they all still had with each other while she felt so distant.

That first night over a big family dinner, everyone chatted animatedly, catching up. Jane tried to join in the conversations but felt like an outsider. All she wanted to do was check her emails in private.

The next few days followed a similar pattern. Jane spent her time isolated on her phone or laptop while everyone else played on the beach, went for bike rides, and cooked meals together. She started feeling depressed, realizing how removed she had become from her family's lives.

On the fourth night, a huge thunderstorm hit, keeping everyone trapped inside. The kids were going stir-crazy, and tempers were starting to flare. Jane's sister Sarah snapped at her for being anti-social and not helping to entertain the kids. Jane snapped back that she didn't sign up for this forced family bonding exercise.

They started yelling at each other, dredging up old grievances and resentments from over the years. Jane's mom started crying, begging them to stop fighting. Jane felt awful for upsetting her mother and ruining the vacation.

She started to walk away, but her dad stopped her, taking her aside. "I know family get-togethers aren't your thing these days. But you've missed so much being away. All your mom and I want is to spend time with our daughter. Please just try, for us?"

Jane softened, suddenly seeing things from their perspective. That night when a board game was suggested, she joined in, helping her niece and nephews with their turns. Laughter and smiles started to return as old rivalries were put aside.

The next day, Jane offered to take her parents out for breakfast, just the three of them. Over pancakes and coffee, they caught up this time, sharing what was going on in their lives beneath the surface. Jane realized how much she had missed them too.

By the end of the vacation, though Jane was beyond ready to get back to work, she felt a weight had been lifted. Reconnecting with her family reminded her that there are things more important in life than a job. She vowed to make more of an effort with them going forward. Maybe forced family vacations weren't so bad after all.

Title: "Strummin' My Heartstrings"

Jenna had always loved music. From a young age, she would spend hours in her bedroom singing along to the radio while strumming her dad's old acoustic guitar. As soon as she was old enough, she decided she wanted to pursue her passion and make a career out of it.

She started by performing at local open mic nights, gradually building up a following in her small hometown. People were impressed with her soulful vocals and heartfelt lyrics. Word spread, and soon she was invited to audition to be the lead singer of an up-and-coming band called "Second Chance."

The first time Jenna met the rest of the band, she instantly clicked with them. They shared the same musical inspirations and vision of making it big one day. The only member she felt slightly intimidated by was their smoldering lead guitarist, Daniel. With his wavy brown hair and leather jacket, he looked like he had stepped right out of a rock poster.

Despite his tough exterior, Daniel truly loved music and poured his heart and soul into his playing. When Jenna heard him perform for the first time, she was awestruck by his raw talent and stage presence. During band practice, she found it hard to take her eyes off him as his fingers flew effortlessly across the fretboard.

Over the next few months, Second Chance started getting more and more gigs as their local fanbase grew. Jenna and Daniel spent hours working on song arrangements together, their musical chemistry undeniable. Off stage, Daniel seemed shy and reserved, but when they played, an unspoken spark passed between them.

One night after a show, some of the band members went out to celebrate at the local bar. Jenna nursed a drink as she watched Daniel chatting with a beautiful blonde down the bar. Feeling melancholy, she soon decided to call it a night, but as she grabbed her coat to leave, Daniel caught up to her.

"Stay, please. I want to talk," he said softly. Jenna's heart pounded as Daniel explained he had felt their connection too but was scared to act on it due to his on-again, off-again relationship. Jenna knew she should walk away to save herself from heartbreak, but being near Daniel was intoxicating. That night, they shared a passionate kiss under the moonlight, and suddenly her silly guitarist crush developed into so much more.

Their fling started cautiously to avoid interfering with the band, but it wasn't long before the rest of Second Chance realized what was going on. Tensions rose as Daniel's girlfriend heard rumors of his infidelity. Jenna worried she was jeopardizing everything they had worked for, but she had truly fallen for Daniel, guitar solos and all.

In the end, following her heart led to more happiness than she ever imagined. Daniel realized his past relationship wasn't meant to be, and he wanted to be with Jenna. Second Chance supported their songwriters, and the band grew stronger than ever. As for Jenna, she finally had her happy ending with the man whose guitar had strummed her heartstrings from day one. Their love song was just beginning.

Title: "A Timely Mistake"

Billy was always fascinated by history and how things came to be. He spent hours in the library researching great discoveries and events from the past. By the age of 12, Billy had already read every book on science and invention they had. That's when he became interested in the idea of time travel.

"Wouldn't it be amazing if we could go back in time and see history unfold for ourselves?" Billy thought. Using his vast knowledge of science, Billy began experimenting with theories on time travel in his bedroom laboratory. After months of tinkering and trial and error, Billy thought he had finally cracked it. He had built a makeshift time machine out of spare parts, wires, and a portable generator.

One sunny Saturday, Billy announced to his parents that he was going to test his invention. "Be careful!" they warned as Billy climbed inside his machine. He pressed the big red button and suddenly felt a whoosh as everything went dark. When Billy opened his eyes, he gasped in amazement. He was no longer in his bedroom - he was standing in a grassy field downtown. But everything looked. Different. The cars were old-fashioned, people wore strange clothing, and there were no cell phones or computers in sight. "It worked!" Billy said in excitement. "I've traveled back in time!"

Billy explored the town, fascinated with everything he saw from a bygone era. As he walked, he noticed a newspaper on the ground announcing the date - September 11, 1901. Billy had traveled back over 100 years! Just then, he spotted a famous inventor working on what looked to be plans for a new airplane. Not thinking, Billy shouted, "You're Orville Wright! Keep working - your first flight will change history!" Orville looked over in surprise at Billy's modern clothes. Had he said too much already?

Later, Billy decided to head back home using his machine. But as he pressed the button, it started sparking and smoking. "No no no!" Billy panicked. The machine had broken down, leaving him stranded over a century in the past. Weeks went by as Billy tried to repair it with limited resources. In the meantime, he supported himself by working odd jobs and doing his schoolwork at the local one-room schoolhouse. The other children treated him as an outcast for his strange knowledge of the future.

One afternoon, Billy was walking near the river when he overheard two men arguing nearby. "Thomas Edison is a fraud! His electric company will never succeed. We must find another way!" said one man. Suddenly, an idea came to Billy. If he changed this moment, it could alter the course of history when he returned to the present. Billy casually stepped in. "Gentlemen, there is a bright future ahead using alternating current. Have you heard of a man named Nikola Tesla...?"

Several months passed as Billy's friendship with Tesla grew. With Billy's knowledge of the future, he helped guide Tesla's ideas, which led to successful developments in AC power that would dominate the industry. Finally, one night there was a breakthrough. Billy had repaired his time machine at last. As he started it up, the town square suddenly lit up all around them. Tesla had succeeded in lighting up the entire town center solely with his alternating current system. The people of the town cheered in amazement. "You did it, my friend. Now go - your work here is done. And thank you for everything." Tesla said, shaking Billy's hand.

In a flash, Billy was transported back to the present. But everything looked...different. Cars flew overhead and there were glowing boxes everywhere that people stared into constantly. Then Billy noticed a history textbook open on his desk. It detailed Nikola Tesla as the most famous and successful inventor in American history, developing groundbreaking technologies that shaped the modern world. Billy gasped as he realized the impact of the changes he had caused in the past. While he was sorry for the mistakes, deep down Billy was glad to have helped the visionary inventor who undoubtedly deserved more credit and success than he previously received in Billy's original timeline. It seems even the smallest moment can have big consequences when traveling through time.

Title: "Nanny or Not Nanny: My Undercover Quest to Take Down a Corrupt Politician"

Jenna had been working as an investigative journalist for 5 years but was starting to feel burnt out on writing the same old stories. She wanted to do an undercover exposé but all of the good stories were already being worked on by other reporters. During a coffee break with her friend Sarah, a new opportunity came up.

"I just saw an ad online looking for a live-in nanny," said Sarah. "Senator Rich is looking for someone to help with his three kids since his wife just took a big job out of the country. Between you and me, there have been some rumors about shady business dealings around his last election campaign. It could be your chance to dig up some dirt!"

Jenna's interest was piqued. She had heard the rumors too but no one had been able to prove anything yet. Going undercover as the nanny could give her unrestricted access to the house and the ability to snoop around after the kids went to bed. "You know, that's not a half-bad idea..." she said slowly as a plan started coming together in her mind.

After an intense weekend of brushing up on her childcare skills and creating a fake resume and references, Jenna landed the nanny job. On her first day, she was surprised by how normal the family seemed. The kids, two boys ages 8 and 6 and a 4-year-old girl, were well-behaved, and the Senator doted on them. Over the next few weeks, she found nothing suspicious in the home or his schedule. Her journalistic instincts told her the dirt must be buried deeper.

One night after the kids were asleep, Jenna heard raised voices coming from the Senator's home office down the hall. Quietly, she crept closer and pressed her ear to the door. "I told you I need another $50,000 by the end of the month or I'm calling the feds," said an angry male voice she didn't recognize. There was some muffled arguing and then the sound of the office door opening. Jenna barely had time to sprint back to the kid's room and pretend to tidy up before the office visitor emerged. She peered through the crack in the door and managed to get a blurry photo of the back of the mystery man's head with her phone.

The next day, Jenna started doing some discrete digging. A quick image search led to a hit—the photo matched Bob Johnson, a known hired gun for local political campaigns. With some social engineering and promises of confidential sources, she was able to get Bob on the phone. At first, he denied anything, but she appealed to his ego, and he started opening up, boasting about his influence. She casually asked what kinds of jobs he had done for the Senator lately. There was a long pause before he said reluctantly, "I shouldn't say anything more." She had her first big lead.

Over the following weeks, Jenna skillfully played both sides, gaining more damning admissions from Bob and documenting questionable expenses on the Senator's books. Just when she thought she had enough for her story, one night she overheard another hushed conversation that revealed an even bigger scheme than she imagined. It was time to bring in the authorities. In a dramatic raid, several high-level arrests were made and hard evidence was seized, all thanks to the intel from one clever nanny. Jenna's exposé rocked the political world and earned her widespread praise. As for her? She was more than ready to get back to writing real news stories, now with a great new chapter added to her resume.

Title: "Feline Rescuer Needs Rescuing"

It was a sunny Saturday afternoon, and the fire station was quiet. John, a 10-year veteran firefighter, was doing some paperwork when the call came in. "Man needs assistance, cat stuck in a tree." John sighed, expecting an easy rescue. These tree cat calls were usually straightforward.

John hopped in the fire truck and headed to the neighborhood where the call was coming from. When he arrived, he saw Bob, a frazzled older man waving his arms frantically from the sidewalk. "Hurry, please help! Fluffy has been up there for hours." John grabbed his harness and climbed up the ladder truck to the lower branches of the large oak tree. Peering up, he spotted a fluffy orange cat perched nervously on a thin limb about 30 feet up.

"Here kitty kitty, it's okay, I've got you," John called out reassuringly. Fluffy meowed pitifully in response. John carefully made his way up through the branches. Finally, he was just below Fluffy and reached out his arms. "Come on boy, jump to daddy." Fluffy hesitated but then leaped into John's waiting arms. "Good boy!" John praised, giving Fluffy a scratch behind the ears to calm him.

But as John turned to begin his descent, there was a loud crack. The branch Fluffy had been on gave way under their combined weight. John and Fluffy tumbled through the air, and John managed to twist at the last second so he took the brunt of the impact against the tree trunk. Both man and cat lay dazed in the branches, uninjured but trapped nearly 40 feet above the ground.

Bob gasped in horror from below. "Oh no, now you're both stuck up there! What do we do?" he cried. John assessed the situation. The branch they had fallen onto was far too thin and fragile to support climbing down. Calling for backup, John radioed for additional engine companies to bring the ladder truck and attempt a rescue.

A half-hour passed with John trying to keep both himself and a now frantic Fluffy calm in the precarious perch. When the backup trucks arrived, firefighters extended the ladder as close as they could get it while still keeping it stable. But it was still 10 feet too short of reaching John and

Fluffy. The firefighters below debated their options, not wanting to risk sending a rescuer up through the unstable tree.

Just then, Fluffy meowed and nudged something towards John - it was a length of rope from his safety harness that had come loose. An idea sparked in John's mind. He tied one end of the rope securely around Fluffy's middle, giving him a few reassuring pets. "Don't worry buddy, I'll get you down safely to your dad." Bob below held out his arms nervously. " lower the cat down slowly," John called down. Hand over hand, John paid out the rope, lowering the bundle of fur into Bob's waiting embrace. Fluffy meowed contentedly, mission accomplished.

One cat was rescued, now for the firefighter. The crews below grasped the end of the rope now anchored around the tree trunk and braced themselves. "Okay, pulling you in slowly now!" they shouted up to John. He tucked in his legs and gripped the rope tightly as his rescuers took up the slack. Slowly, painfully slowly, he felt himself being lowered toward the ground as the branches grabbed and tugged at his uniform. Finally, with a whoosh and a cheer, John's boots hit solid earth. Fluffy meowed and head-butted his leg in thanks. John smiled down at the feline. "Just doing my job to help those in need, furry or not. Now, who's up for some tuna?"

Title: "Mayday Mayday, This is Flight 642 Requesting Emergency Landing"

Captain Sarah Jones gripped the control yoke tightly as the engine on her small passenger plane sputtered and died. "Mayday Mayday, this is Flight 642, we have lost our number one engine and are requesting emergency landing clearance immediately." She kept her voice calm but inside her heart was racing.

She glanced over at her co-pilot Brad, who was even paler than usual. Brad was just 6 months out of flight school, and this was only his second trip in the right seat. His hands were clenched together so tight his knuckles were turning white. "It's going to be okay Brad, I've landed much bigger planes in worse conditions than this. Just stay calm and help me run through the checklists."

Brad nodded but didn't look very reassured. Sarah could understand why he was nervous; losing an engine was never part of the plan, but she had complete confidence in her abilities. She just needed Brad to hold it together so they could get their 12 passengers down safely. Air traffic control came back, advising they had the airport in sight and was clearing the runway for their emergency landing.

"Alright Brad, I'm going to need you to focus. Call out the checklist items and I'll complete them. The more methodical we are about this, the smoother the landing will be." Brad shakily started calling out the pre-landing flow, and Sarah efficiently worked through securing the cabin and engine. Without the power of two engines, they'd have to lose some altitude on the glide slope, which would require perfect timing of flaps, spoilers, and throttle control.

As they descended on the final approach, Brad's voice got higher and reedier with each checklist item. Sarah knew he was barely holding it together but didn't have time to coddle him right now. She focused completely on lining up with the runway, adjusting pitch and power exactly as needed to maintain the 3-degree descent path. The touchdown came smoothly, right at the beginning of the runway given their reduced performance. Sarah reversed the thrust and applied maximum braking to bring the aircraft to a full stop safely at the far end.

She taxied to the nearest terminal, shut down the remaining engine, and let out a long sigh. Turning to Brad, who had both hands clapped over his mouth trying not to be sick, she said, "You did great up there. Not everyone keeps it together that well on their second emergency. Why don't you go check on the passengers, and I'll finish up the shutdown paperwork? You'll be landing like a pro in no time."

Brad managed a queasy smile. "I don't know about that, but thanks for getting us down in one piece Captain. You are as good as they say." He unbuckled shakily and headed back to reassure the passengers. Sarah smiled, glad she could keep both her co-pilot and the passengers calm in a crisis. It was all part of the job, but sometimes having a natural talent for staying cool under pressure came in handy. Just another day in the life of a pilot.

Title: "Funny Man at the Funeral"

Jerry was a well-known stand-up comedian who was always the life of the party. However, one day he got a call that would be one of the toughest gigs of his career - he was asked to tell some jokes and try to lighten the mood at his old friend Bob's funeral. Jerry thought they must be joking at first, but they assured him the family thought it was what Bob would have wanted.

The day of the funeral arrived, and Jerry struggled to come up with anything funny. As he sat in the church looking out at all the mournful faces, he began to doubt this was a good idea. But then it was his turn to speak. He slowly walked up to the podium and cleared his throat.

"So... I bet you're all wondering why they asked a comedian to speak at a funeral," he began. A few people let out nervous laughs. "Well, Bob was one of my oldest and dearest friends. He loved to laugh more than anyone I knew. One time we were at a party and Bob accidentally spilled his beer all down the front of this guy he didn't even know! The look on the guy's face was priceless. Of course, Bob apologized like crazy but he couldn't stop laughing about it either."

Jerry told a few more stories that helped the congregation remember Bob's fun-loving spirit through smiles instead of just tears. By the end, people were drying their eyes but with laughter instead of just sorrow. Jerry looked out at the family's appreciative faces, feeling like he made his friend proud one last time. Even in death, Bob found a way to bring a little humor and light to an otherwise somber occasion. Jerry realized sometimes even in our grief, laughter truly is the best medicine.

Title: "Pixel Crush: My VR Date with Destiny"

Jimmy was the biggest gamer you ever saw. Every night after school, he would rush home and log countless hours in his favorite VR MMORPG, saving the kingdom of Gamelandia from the forces of evil. Through all his adventures, one player stood out to him - the mighty warrior princess knew only as "XoXoGamerGurlXoXo".

Though they had never met IRL, Jimmy felt a real connection with GamerGurl as they battled side by side. Her lightning-fast reflexes and insightful strategies complemented his strength and resilience perfectly. Together, their duo was simply unstoppable. Jimmy found himself thinking of her even when he wasn't logged on.

One day, Jimmy saw a commercial for a big cash prize VR gaming tournament happening in the city. He knew this was his chance to finally meet his pixel crush IRL! After much practicing, Jimmy made it through the qualifying rounds to the finals. The championship came down to a one-on-one duel between Jimmy and none other than GamerGurl herself!

As their avatars faced off, Jimmy's heart was pounding. But when GamerGurl's avatar glitched briefly, revealing her IRL self on the other side, Jimmy gasped. GamerGurl was his longtime neighbor and crush, Jessica! Jessica smiled back, clearly also surprised but happy.

In the excitement of the reveal, both players lost focus and were defeated by another finalist. But they didn't care about the prize - they had found something even better that day. From that moment on, their adventure continued not just in VR...but in real life too. The end!

Title: "Houston, We Have a Problem: How Sally Saved the Day"

Sally sighed as she looked out the window of the space shuttle at the vast emptiness of space. It had been a long 6 months away from Earth and she was ready to come home. But first, she had one last job to do - inspect the exterior of the shuttle for any damage or problems before beginning their re-entry.

She suited up and went through the airlock, clutching her space walk tether tightly. As she made her way slowly around the shuttle, she noticed something wasn't right with one of the heat shields. Upon closer inspection, she realized with horror that it had somehow come loose during their journey.

"Houston, this is Sally. We have a major problem," she radioed down. "Heat shield six is detached. I'm going to try to secure it but I'm worried it won't hold for re-entry. Any ideas?"

The response from mission control was grim. "Sally, without that heat shield intact, the temperatures on re-entry will be off the charts in that area. It's likely the shuttle will break apart. Do you have the materials and tools up there to attempt a repair?"

Sally's heart sank. If she couldn't fix it, she and her crew were doomed. But she wasn't ready to give up yet. "Let me take a look in the supply closet and I'll get back to you," she responded, trying to keep the panic out of her voice so as not to worry the others.

Floating weightlessly in the microgravity of the shuttle, Sally rummaged through the closet. Duct tape, zip ties, welding supplies - surely something could work! Then an idea came to her. She gathered up a roll of industrial strength tape, extra rolls of repair fabric, and the caulk gun. Time to get to work.

Out in the vacuum again, Sally made her way back to the damaged heat shield. The first step was cleaning and prepping the surface so the tape and fabric would stick properly. Sweat beaded on her forehead inside her helmet as the sunshine-like heat of space warmed her through the insulated suit.

After what felt like hours of careful sanding, wiping down with solvent, and letting everything dry, it was time for the repairs to begin.

Rolling out the longest piece of tape she could get, Sally stretched it across the damaged area, hoping it would hold. Next, she layered strips of the repair fabric on top, smoothing them down and packing them in tight with her gloved hands. Finally, she caulked over the whole thing, sealing and reinforcing the patch. Step by excruciating step, she worked to salvage their ride home.

By the time Sally radioed down again, she was beyond exhausted. But she had good news. "Patch is complete. How does it look from down there?" she asked Mission Control. The response was overwhelmingly positive - from the satellite images, it appeared her makeshift repair job had done the trick. They gave her the all-clear for re-entry.

Cheers erupted over the radio as Sally made her way wearily back inside. Her crewmates enveloped her in hugs, beyond grateful for her quick thinking and bravery under pressure. As their shuttle began its blazing descent back through the atmosphere, Sally smiled with relief and satisfaction. She had saved the day with little more than tape and caulk. Just another day in the life of an astronaut, she thought with a chuckle. Another story to tell when she finally made it home.

Title: "A Deadline to Meet"

John rubbed his tired eyes as he stared at the blank Word document on his computer screen. As a freelance writer, he was used to tight deadlines but this took the cake. One week to write a 50,000-word novel? It would be impossible for most people. But John had a family to support and bills to pay so he didn't have a choice.

He brewed his fifth cup of coffee of the day and took a sip, hoping the caffeine would give his fried brain the boost it needed. But after hours of staring, not a single word had been written. John was starting to worry he'd let down his publisher and all the people depending on him.

Just then, John's daughter Sarah peeked into the office. "Daddy, why are you still working? Come watch a movie with me and mum!" she said with her usual bright smile. How John wished he could join them but he had to find a way to make progress.

"I'm sorry sweetie, Daddy has to write a big book for work. How about you pick out the movie and I'll come see the start of it before bed?" John replied gently. Sarah nodded understandingly and skipped away. Her smile gave John the strength to keep going despite his exhaustion.

He opened up a new document and started typing, "Chapter 1". But just then, the family's elderly neighbor Mrs. Johnson knocked on the door. "Sorry to bother you dearly, but my fence blew over in the storm. Do you think you could help me repair it tomorrow?" she asked hopefully. John couldn't say no to her sweet face.

"Of course Mrs. Johnson, I'll come by first thing. For now, though, let me walk you home safely." John smiled and grabbed his coat. As they strolled together down the dark street lit only by lampposts, Mrs. Johnson told John funny stories from her childhood that took his mind off his deadline worries for a while. She had a way of finding humor even in hard times.

When John finally returned home, he noticed Sarah had fallen asleep on the couch during the movie. He carried her gently to bed and tucked her in, kissing her on the forehead. "Goodnight darling. Daddy loves you," he whispered. Seeing his daughter's peaceful face filled John's heart with warmth and reminded him of why this deadline was so important.

Renewed with determination, John sat back down to write. The memories of Mrs. Johnson's laughter and Sarah's smile inspired him. Suddenly, the words began flowing from his fingertips like a river. He wrote long into the night, stopping only to refill his coffee. By morning sunlight, John leaned back with a satisfied sigh. 50,000 words stared back at him from the screen - his completed novel, done with a day to spare.

He sent the file off to his publisher, wondering what new adventures this story of family, friendship, and humor would bring its readers. As for John, it was time for a well-deserved sleep with dreams of many more books to come. His family and neighborhood friends would always give him the strength to beat any deadline.

Title: "A Royal Feast to Remember"

Sophia couldn't believe it when she got the call. The Head Chef of the Royal Palace had fallen ill, and they needed a temporary replacement to cook for the King's birthday feast in just three days. As one of the top private chefs in the country, she had been recommended. How could she turn down such a prestigious opportunity, even if it was extremely short notice?

She spent the next 48 hours in a flurry of activity. Reviewed the detailed menu plan that had been prepared, making lists of all the ingredients she would need to purchase, and practicing each dish to perfection. On the morning of the feast, she loaded up her van and made the two-hour drive to the palace, nerves already starting to kick in.

She was shown to the enormous palace kitchen, bigger than any restaurant she had ever worked in. Dozens of other chefs were also busy at work, preparing sides and finishing touches for the hundred guests that would be attending. Sophia got to work, dicing, slicing, and sautéing with laser focus. She wanted this meal to be perfect.

A few hours before service, the Head Butler came in to check on progress. "Everything is looking wonderful so far, Chef. His Majesty will be most pleased, I'm sure. Oh, and a word of warning, the Prince has decided he wants to help in the kitchen this evening. Try not to let him underfoot too much!"

Sure enough, not long after, a young man popped his head in the kitchen. "Hello all! I'm Prince Charles, how can I lend a hand?" The staff politely found the Prince trivial tasks to keep him occupied, while Sophia continued overseeing the cooking of the main courses.

As the first guests began arriving, Sophia did final taste tests and decided everything was ready. "Service!" She called out, and the kitchen swung into action. Plating each dish with artistic flair and speedily passing them off to the waiting staff.

The first few courses went off without a hitch, and Sophia started to relax, growing more confident in the kitchen of the Royal Family. But then disaster struck - one of the kitchen helpers accidentally knocked over a pot of boiling stock right as Prince Charles was walking by. The scalding liquid spilled all down the front of his formal attire. Chaos erupted as people rushed to help the Prince.

Thinking fast, Sophia corralled two chefs. "You, go find some spare clothes for His Highness. And you, start reheating these entrées right away, we can't delay service." Once the Prince was rushed off to change, she turned back to the stove. "Alright team, we've got this, let's get these meals back on track!"

By some miracle, they managed to get the food relaunched with only a 10-minute delay. The night continued without further mishaps. As the guests polished off the final dessert course, Sophia sagged against the counter in relief that her role in the royal feast was over.

A few days later, she received a personal thank-you letter from Prince Charles himself, praising her calm handling of the kitchen emergency. It turned out the King had also heard of her talents through the grapevine. A few months down the road, Sophia accepted the full-time position of Head Royal Chef. It seems one little mishap was all it took for her big culinary break. To this day, that feast remains the most memorable of her career.

Title: "Riding the Monster Wave"

Johnny couldn't believe his eyes when he saw the massive wave approaching on the horizon. All the other surfers were heading back to shore, but something told Johnny this was his chance. Ever since he was a young boy, all he wanted to do was take on the biggest waves. While others feared what lay beyond the break, for Johnny, facing the unknown is what living was all about.

Gripping his surfboard tightly, Johnny paddled with all his might to position himself just right. This wave was unlike anything he had ever seen before. It must have been 100 feet tall! His heart was racing as the wave began to crest. With perfect timing, Johnny popped up to his feet and began carving down the face of the watery mountain. The power of the wave was unreal. Johnny felt as if he was flying.

For a few brief seconds, it seemed Johnny had tamed the monster. But then, without warning, the wave suddenly broke and Johnny found himself overwhelmed by the massive volume of water. He fought to get up for air but the force was too great. Just when he thought it was over, Johnny felt a strong hand grab him and yank him upwards. Through the water rushing past, he saw it was his friend Mike who had paddled out to rescue him, at great risk to himself.

Coughing and gasping, Johnny collapsed on his board as Mike helped paddle them back to safety. As they reached the shore, all the other surfers cheered wildly for Johnny's brave but nearly tragic ride. From that day on, Johnny was a hero in the surfing community for having the courage and skill to battle the biggest wave anyone had ever seen. But for Johnny, he knew it was thanks to his true friend Mike that he lived to surf another day.

Title: "A Lesson in Likes"

Mrs. Johnson had lived next door to the Smith family for over 30 years. At 85 years old, she enjoyed her quiet routine of gardening, baking cookies, and sitting on her front porch watching the neighborhood go by.

One summer evening, 10-year-old Tommy Smith was outside playing catch with his dad when he noticed Mrs. Johnson staring longingly at their iPhone as they scrolled through photos on Facebook. "Dad, I think Mrs. Johnson wants to learn about our phones," Tommy said.

Being the kind boy he was, Tommy asked Mrs. Johnson if she'd like to learn about social media. "All the kids are on it these days, I feel so left out not knowing what it's all about!" she admitted. And so began Tommy's lessons.

Every afternoon after school, Tommy would head next door and show Mrs. Johnson something new on his iPhone. He walked her through the basics of Facebook - how to create a profile, add friends, and post statuses, and photos. Mrs. Johnson was enthralled looking at pictures her friends and family had shared from around the world.

Tommy then introduced Instagram and showed her how to post a photo from the app of her homemade oatmeal cookies. "Now people can see what a great baker you are!" he said. Within an hour, the post had over a dozen likes. Mrs. Johnson was tickled pink that her cooking was getting such a positive response online.

Their sessions continued with Mrs. Johnson quickly gaining more followers and liking others' posts too. Tommy taught her how to post selfies, give comments, and use hashtags to engage more on social media. One day, a video chat request came through on Facebook - it was Mrs. Johnson's granddaughter calling from Australia!

"Tommy, I can't thank you enough for your patience and for teaching me these new skills. I feel so connected to being able to see what everyone is up to each day. You've helped bring me into the modern world!" Mrs. Johnson gushed. As a thank you, she began baking double batches of cookies to share with the Smith family.

Word spread through the neighborhood about Tommy's lessons. Soon other elderly neighbors were lining up at Mrs. Johnson's porch to get their tech tutorials. Tommy happily shared his knowledge with all. It warmed his heart to see the joy technology was bringing to the older generation. He had a feeling this was the start of strong new bonds and friendships throughout the community.

Title: "A Family's Love"

Joe and Mary were driving back to their childhood home after receiving a call from their father that their mother had taken a turn for the worse in her battle with cancer. Pulling up the long driveway, memories of their times growing up on the farm came flooding back.

As they entered the house, they found their parents in the living room. Their father John looked exhausted as he cared for his wife Sarah around the clock. When Sarah saw her children, she broke into a smile which quickly turned into a fit of coughing. Joe and Mary rushed to her side, patting her back until the coughing subsided.

That night over a subdued dinner, John explained the doctor's prognosis wasn't good and Sarah may only have a few weeks left. Choking back tears, he said he wasn't sure how much longer he could manage on his own. Joe and Mary assured their dad they would both move back home to share the load.

The next morning, Joe and Mary began to argue over the best way to care for their mother. Mary felt Joe was too brusque in his manner while assisting Sarah while Joe thought Mary fussed too much. Their raised voices could be heard throughout the house. When John told them to keep it down for fear of upsetting Sarah, they both sheepishly apologized.

Realizing their bickering wasn't helping anyone, that afternoon Joe and Mary sat down to have a heart-to-heart. Through tears, they acknowledged how difficult this was for both of them but said what was most important now was being there for their parents. They agreed to divvy up responsibilities so one could spell the other as needed.

In the following weeks, through working as a team, Joe and Mary found a routine that worked. Most importantly, their presence lifted their parents' spirits. On one of Sarah's last days, she clasped Joe and Mary's hands and smiled, saying she was at peace knowing they would all be okay and continue to support each other. A few days later, surrounded by her loving family, Sarah passed away peacefully.

While grief lingered heavily in their hearts, Joe, Mary, and John took comfort that in Sarah's final chapter, her children had put aside their differences to come together and give their mother the care she deserved. Their selfless acts of compassion ensured their parents' final days had been filled with love, laughter, and family - the most anyone in her place could ask for.

Title: "A Helping Paw and a New Lease on Life"

John was always a shy person. He dreaded any kind of public speaking and avoided large crowds whenever possible. His job as an accountant allowed him to work mostly alone in a small office, which suited him just fine.

One weekend, John decided to get away from the city for a bit of quiet relaxation. He packed a bag and drove a few hours to a more rural area, planning to explore some parks and hiking trails. As he walked along a wooded path, enjoying the solitude, he spotted some movement out of the corner of his eye. Moving closer, he saw a small dog limping badly in the underbrush.

The dog was whimpering in pain, unable to put weight on one of its front legs. John crouched down slowly so as not to startle it. "Hey buddy, it's okay. I'm not going to hurt you." He spoke softly and extended his hand for the dog to sniff. After a moment of hesitating, the dog limped over and sniffed John's hand, seemingly reassured.

John examined the leg gently. It was broken. He needed to get the dog help right away but was worried about moving it. After thinking for a moment, he took off his jacket and made a makeshift sling. Sliding the jacket under the dog, he lifted it carefully into his arms. The dog yelped in pain but settled against John's chest, seeming to understand he was being helped.

Carrying the injured dog, John rushed back to his car and sped toward the nearest veterinary clinic. The vet took one look at the dog's swollen leg and rushed it back for X-rays. John paced in the waiting room for over an hour before the vet finally reemerged.

"The good news is, it's a clean break," she told John. "We were able to set the leg and put on a cast. With some medication and rest, he should heal up just fine. The not-so-good news is, he's a stray with no owner. The shelter is full up so they can't take him. Are you able to foster him until his leg heals and he's adoptable?"

John was taken aback by the request. He had never had a pet before due to his shy nature. But the memory of that poor dog limping in pain and trusting him for help tugged at his heartstrings. "Well...I guess he can stay with me until he's better." John agreed.

And so Diego, as John had decided to name the dog, came home with him. At first, John still felt awkward taking care of an animal, but Diego seemed grateful just to have a comfortable place to rest. Within a few days, John found himself looking forward to feeding Diego, changing his bandages, and giving him gentle belly rubs when the medication made him drowsy. Diego's cheerful but calm demeanor started to rub off on John.

As the weeks went by and Diego's leg began to heal, John found himself more at ease around the friendly dog. Diego seemed to sense when John was feeling shy or nervous and would nuzzle up next to him on the couch until John started to relax and pet him. One day, John realized with a start that he was no longer dreading the return to work after his weekend away. He was starting to think he might even enjoy interacting with people more now.

Finally, the day came when Diego had his cast removed. The vet gave him a clean bill of health and said he was ready to be adopted. John was proud of how far Diego had come, but also sad at the thought of saying goodbye to his canine companion. That's when the vet had another suggestion - why didn't John adopt Diego himself?

"I think you two have bonded over these past months," she said. "Diego loves you and you've become more comfortable around him. It would be a shame to separate you now." John thought about it and realized the vet was right. He had grown quite fond of Diego during their time together. With Diego by his side, John no longer felt so shy or nervous about trying new things.

And so Diego officially became a part of John's family. John even started volunteering at the local animal shelter on weekends, helping other dogs find homes just as Diego had found his. Thanks to helping one little dog in need, John had found not only a loyal canine companion but also a new sense of purpose and confidence in himself. His shyness was now a thing of the past.

Title: "When Grandma Gets a Handmade Gift"

Grandma Jane was in the kitchen baking banana bread for her weekly book club meeting. The smell was wafting through the house as her grandchildren Timmy and Sally were playing upstairs.

Jane was just taking the bread out of the oven when she heard little footsteps running down the stairs. "Grandma, Grandma, we made you something!" shouted Timmy as he burst into the kitchen, Sally right behind him.

"Oh my, what did you make for me?" asked Grandma with a smile, wiping her hands on her apron. Timmy proudly held out a large piece of paper with lots of colorful scribbles all over it. "We made you a picture!" he said.

Grandma took the paper and looked it over. "Hmm, let me see. I see a big yellow circle, that must be the sun. And here are some green trees. Oh! And is this me and you playing in the backyard?" she asked, pointing to two stick figures.

"Yeah!" said Timmy excitedly. "And here is our dog Spot." Grandma examined the brown blob Timmy was referring to. "Well, it's a lovely picture boy. I just love all the bright colors. Thank you so much!" She gave each of them a big hug.

"That's not all Grandma," said Sally. "I made you something too with Ms. Johnson at school." She proudly held out a lumpy blue object. Grandma examined it quizzically. "What is this?" she asked. "It's a homemade vase for your flowers!" Sally explained.

Grandma could see now that it was meant to hold flowers. The sides were uneven, and there was a bumpy texture to it from Sally's small fingers pressing and shaping the wet clay. But it warmed Grandma's heart to see her grandchildren putting so much care and thought into gifts for her, even if they weren't perfect.

"It's absolutely beautiful Sally, I love it. And look, I just happen to have some daisies from the garden that will look lovely in it." Grandma arranged the white flowers in the vase and placed them in the center of the kitchen table. "Now we have something handmade from each of you to enjoy. I'll treasure these always."

That Saturday, Grandma's book club was coming over for their weekly meeting and cookies. As the ladies filed into the kitchen, they all stopped to admire the picture on the refrigerator and the homemade vase of flowers on the table.

"Jane, these are just precious. Did your grandchildren make these for you?" asked Betty. "They sure did. Aren't they so thoughtful and creative?" beamed Grandma. The other ladies all agreed on what special gifts they were.

Just then, Timmy and Sally came bounding down the stairs, wanting to say hi to all the ladies. "Oh, come look at what else Sally made for me in art class today!" said Grandma. She pulled a piece of paper out of her pocket with a funny stick figure drawing on it. All the ladies "oohed" and "aahed" over it, making Sally grin from ear to ear.

Grandma knew just how to encourage her grandchildren's imaginations and appreciate their little creations, even if they weren't perfect. And it warmed her heart each time they presented her with another gift, no matter how lumpy or misshapen. Because with each one came a big reminder of how much they cared for their Grandma.

www.ingramcontent.com/pod-product-compliance
Lightning Source LLC
Chambersburg PA
CBHW082136290526
45794CB00008B/3062